W9-CON-473

PERSPECTIVES ON AIDS

Ethical
and
Social
Issues

Christine Overall, Editor
with
William P. Zion, Associate Editor

Toronto Oxford New York
OXFORD UNIVERSITY PRESS

Oxford University Press, 70 Wynford Drive, Don Mills, Ontario M3C 1J9

Toronto Oxford New York
Delhi Bombay Calcutta Madras Kuala Lumpur
Singapore Hong Kong Tokyo Nairobi Dar es Salaam
Cape Town Melbourne Auckland Madrid

and associated companies in
Berlin Ibadan

Dedication

For the Re-Evaluation Counseling Communities of Ontario (C.O.)

In memory of J.W. and J.G. (W.Z.)

RC607
.A26P475
1991

Photograph credits:
Figures: 1 and 2, Courtesy *Weekly World News*.
3, By Sandra Peplar, courtesy of *The Anglican Magazine*.
4, Courtesy of the artist, David Horsley. 5, Courtesy of
the artist, André Durand.

CANADIAN CATALOGUING IN PUBLICATION DATA
Main entry under title:
Perspectives on AIDS : ethical and social issues
Includes bibliographical references and index.
ISBN 0-19-540749-0
1. AIDS (Disease) – Social aspects.
2. AIDS (Disease) – Moral and ethical aspects. I. Overall,
Christine, 1949– . II. Zion, William P.
RC607.A26P47 1991   362.1'969792   C91-093127-5

Copyright © Christine Overall and William Zion 1991
OXFORD is a trademark of Oxford University Press
2 3 4 5 – 95 94 93 92
Designed by Heather Delfino
Printed in Canada by Gagné Printing Ltd.

CONTENTS

ACKNOWLEDGEMENTS

We wish to thank Richard Teleky, our editor at Oxford University Press, for his patience, support, and commitment throughout the preparation of this volume and Sally Livingston, our copy editor, for her thorough and careful work. We are also grateful for the assistance of the staff of the Kingston AIDS Project, particularly Blair Collins and Nancy Tatham.

Christine Overall thanks Ann Liblik and Jackie Doherty for their hard work and their encouragement, and Ted, Devon, and Narnia Worth for their love and lightheartedness. She also thanks the members of the Re-Evaluation Communities of Kingston, Toronto, and Ottawa, particularly Blair Voyvodic and Bruce Small, for their leadership and their optimism.

William Zion thanks Robert Henderson and Andrew Taylor for the stimulating dialogue, and Rhoda for her support.

INTRODUCTION

In mid-1990, an ominous-sounding slogan appeared on billboards in Toronto: 'AIDS: Stick it in your head instead!'[1] The threatening tone of the message, its not-so-subtle sexual undertones, and the fact that it resulted from a bungled translation of an idiomatic French slogan are ironically emblematic of the contemporary culture of the so-called 'AIDS crisis'. Acquired Immunodeficiency Syndrome (AIDS) is a condition that often occasions tremendous fear; it is closely associated with sexuality; and it is more misunderstood and misinterpreted than understood.[2]

Why has AIDS been, and why does it continue to be, a particularly problematic and frightening issue? First, of course, because it is potentially deadly. While the debate continues about possible 'co-factors', the cause of AIDS, discovered in 1985, is the Human Immunodeficiency Virus (HIV), a constantly mutating retrovirus that gradually destroys the T-cells that protect the body against infections. In the final stage of HIV infection, AIDS proper, the body is unable to resist so-called 'opportunistic diseases' such as Kaposi's sarcoma and pneumocistis carinii pneumonia (PCP). So the awareness of AIDS brings out people's deepest fears about illness, disability, and their own mortality.

Second, no cure for HIV infection has yet been discovered, and although some drugs are being used to slow the spread of the virus and to stave off serious infections, no effective vaccine has yet been created. These facts may occasion a kind of atavistic fear of nature gone wild. They confront human beings with the limits of human control, and with the realization that, despite what the media may encourage us to think, the scientific enterprise is not infallible.

Third, HIV infection is spreading rapidly. In Canada, as of mid-1990, 3,818 cases of AIDS have been reported, and of these 2,282 (59 per cent) have died. Although national statistics on HIV infection are not reported in Canada, the use of a blood test that reveals the presence of antibodies to the virus has revealed that many thousands more are infected, or HIV-positive. The Federal

Centre for AIDS predicts as many as 12,890 cases of AIDS in Canada by 1993; indeed, the number of reported cases is currently doubling every twenty-five months. Worldwide, as of May 1990, about 228,874 people had been reported with AIDS.[3] Thus many of those who write about AIDS use the term 'epidemic' to describe it, and many have talked about the similarities between this infection and epidemics of the past.

Fourth, apart from the HIV-antibody test, it is not always possible to tell who is a carrier of this infection. Although those with fully developed AIDS may be very ill, persons in the early stages of infection, who are carriers of HIV, can be asymptomatic for months or even years before becoming ill. This fact may foster much of the current confusion and inconsistency in many people's thinking about the transmission of HIV. For example, although transmission of the virus occurs only through the exchange of bodily fluids such as semen, vaginal fluids, blood, or breast milk, many still believe, erroneously, that infection can occur by almost magical means – that is, by casual everyday contact. At the same time, paradoxically, there is insufficient understanding of the real risks of activities such as sharing needles during drug use, or engaging in high-risk unprotected sexual activities such as oral, vaginal, or anal intercourse. Many who are vulnerable to AIDS not only remain unprotected but continue in behaviour that places them in constant danger of HIV infection. Denial and negation remain primary defences against the knowledge that AIDS can afflict anyone.

Fifth, since HIV can be transmitted through some sexual activities, it has become associated with what are loosely and unthinkingly called 'promiscuity' and 'deviance', and with the negative moral judgements attendant on these terms.[4] Despite lip-service to supposed 'sexual liberation', Canadians are still not very open, flexible, or clear-thinking about sexual practices, and sexual behaviour continues to be an area of particular fear, coercion, and confusion in people's lives.

The very nature of HIV infection as a breakdown of the immune system, leaving the body subject to opportunistic infections, lends itself to a mystique. Even seemingly objective presentations of AIDS by researchers such as Robert Gallo and Peter Jaret abound in metaphors of invasion, of wars between good and evil, and of modern communication systems.[5] Linking this kind of language to that used for sexuality produces a potent combination – even physicians often indulge in talk about guilty and innocent 'victims of AIDS'. Just as, in the recent past, language about 'venereal' disease was rarely free of metaphors of shame, dirt, and guilt, so AIDS inherits a legacy of sexual prudery and prurience, anxiety and homophobia (the fear and hatred of homosexuals). In the social response to epidemics of the past, sexuality, impurity, and disease have often been linked: where disease is thought to be the consequence of sexual 'sin', illness is constructed in terms of exclusion and inclusion, structural impurity versus the purity of those who are 'clean'. That this culture has not educated people carefully and openly about which activities are dangerous, about the use and availability of condoms, about the prevalence of homosexuality and the dangers of needle-sharing, shows that the fears about sex and death associated with past epidemics still permeate the present.

Sixth, AIDS involves groups that are already the target of stigmatization in this culture. Much contemporary AIDS discourse is laden with images and metaphors of evil outsiders – gay men, people of colour, prostitutes, intravenous drug-users – introducing the lethal virus into the community of the righteous, the straight, and the clean. Entire groups of people are stigmatized and treated as separate from the supposedly distinct and more valuable 'general population'. The exclusion of marginalized members of society and the perception of AIDS as a disease that reveals their hidden identity as deviants brings a false sense of security to a threatened society.

AIDS was first defined as GRID, or 'Gay Related Immunodeficiency Syndrome'; it has often been described in the popular media as the 'gay plague', and it continues to be thought of, mistakenly, as the disease of gay men. The long association, in the popular imagination, between 'unnatural' sexual practices and the Devil, together with the fact that buggery was listed as a crime in traditional common law, to a large degree provides the foundation for the uncaring, if not antagonistic, attitude of many towards persons living with AIDS. But although 79 per cent of people with AIDS in Canada have been infected through homosexual or bisexual activity,[6] increasing numbers of heterosexual adults of both sexes, as well as children not yet sexually active, are also infected with HIV. Although the bearers of infection are often falsely imagined to be 'outsiders', HIV does not discriminate among those it infects.

Perspectives on AIDS: Ethical and Social Issues is a collection of essays by Canadian academics and activists who explore some difficult questions relating to AIDS and HIV infection in North America, particularly within the context of Canadian culture and the Canadian health-care system. As these papers demonstrate, AIDS and HIV infection have become the focus of a continuing tension between care for individuals and concern for the various communities of which those individuals are members. Addressing the ethical and social problems raised by AIDS requires consideration of questions about individual and collective rights, about autonomy and informed consent, and about non-maleficence, or the avoidance of harm, in personal relationships, health care, education, and social policy. Equally important, it requires an awareness of the social and political dimensions of HIV infection: the cultural construction of AIDS language, images, and representations; the pervasive effects of racism and homophobia; the scapegoating and marginalization of groups such as gays, prostitutes, and intravenous drug users; the oppression of women; and the power and authority of the medical and scientific establishments.

The anthology is divided into two sections. The first, 'Culture and Context', examines some of the social parameters that define perceptions of HIV infection within Canadian culture. It poses questions about the harmful effects of the dominant values, language, and images that construct current understandings of AIDS, and challenges their appropriateness and justification. 'AIDS: The Social Dimension', by Arthur Schafer, suggests that some central values in Canadian society, values such as rationality, altruism, public-spiritedness, and a sense of humanity, are being attenuated by current responses to AIDS. These responses encourage the scapegoating of individuals believed to be at fault for being HIV-infected; they foster xenophobia (fear and hatred of 'outsiders'); they compromise the development of critical thinking; and they promote an emphasis on self-interest at the expense of public-spiritedness. In these ways AIDS poses a challenge not only to life and health, but to significant moral values.

In 'AIDS and Disability' Jerome E. Bickenbach outlines an innovative social context for responding to HIV infection. He shows that having AIDS or being HIV-infected is both a physical disability (a medical condition) and a physical handicap (a sociological or political category): a disabling physical condition that has also become a social disadvantage through stigmatization and discrimination. He argues that a disability-rights framework provides a helpful and fair context for the adjudication of conflicts – between the rights of persons who are HIV-positive and those who are not infected, and between effective public health measures and the sacrifices demanded by those measures from individual citizens. Such a framework would give appropriate recognition to the fact that persons who are HIV-positive constitute a vulnerable minority, who are entitled to consideration equal to that given to persons who are not infected.

In most current social responses to AIDS, women have continued to constitute a neglected minority. In 'AIDS and Women: The (Hetero)Sexual Politics of HIV Infection', Christine Overall discusses some ways in which cultural interpretations of and reactions to AIDS reflect attitudes and practices that are oppressive to women, particularly in the vulnerable areas of sexuality and procreation: through the entrenchment of gender stereotypes; through the exacerbation of inequality between women and men; and through the uncritical acceptance of ideas about the 'essential' natures of males and females and of heterosexuals and homosexuals. Thus HIV infection constitutes for women, as for gay men, not only a serious medical condition but also a threatening political problem.

Investigation of the metaphors by which AIDS is currently being interpreted, of their hidden meanings and their plausibility, is the only means by which they may be purged. From within the religious traditions, alternative approaches to understanding AIDS are explored by William Zion in 'AIDS, Ethics and Religion'. He shows that the interpretation of AIDS as a punishment for sexual sin is a misreading of the Jewish and Christian traditions.

Alternatively, recognition of the link between Christ and the suffering, and acceptance of homosexuals as persons whose relationships can be loving and responsible, provides a way to move beyond traditional religious homophobia. A critique of homophobic traditions, their roots and sources, is vital if persecution of persons living with AIDS (PLWAS, or PWAS) is to cease.

The idea of the 'victim' of AIDS, a graphic metaphor vigorously rejected by AIDS activists, dominates much current popular writing about HIV infection. This 'victim' is constructed simultaneously as sinner and saint, since AIDS is imagined to originate in sexual sin and to issue in a death that is viewed as both punishment and apotheosis. James Miller's ironically titled paper, 'Acquired Immanent Divinity Syndrome', explores the representation of persons living with AIDS as late-twentieth-century martyrs, both within conservative political doctrines and within the countercultural ethos of AIDS activism. Miller shows the terrible ambiguity that lies in the glorification of the sinner/saint, which is the legacy of Christianity.

The second section of this book, 'Ethical and Social Issues', probes some specific questions about rights and freedoms, care and liberation, both for those who are and for those who are not HIV-infected. The unifying theme of these papers is the concern for and commitment to the promotion of self-determination, particularly for those who have AIDS or are HIV-positive. In 'Sexual Ethics and AIDS: A Liberal View', Michael Yeo examines some questions about sexual responsibility, sexual freedom, and sexual behaviour in an era when certain sexual acts may be the occasion for transmission of HIV. Setting aside questions about the 'naturalness' or 'normality' of sexual activities, the paper uses informed consent as the central moral criterion for evaluating sexual behaviour. Yeo argues that sexual responsibility should be assessed with regard to a 'standard of disclosure' of information designed to promote informed consent of prospective partners to sexual activities.

Benjamin Freedman discusses a central question about HIV infection with respect to health-care workers such as physicians and nurses: what is the basis for and the extent of their obligations to their patients? In 'Health-Care Workers' Occupational Exposure to HIV: Obligations and Entitlements', Freedman argues that health-care workers have a moral obligation to care for those with AIDS or HIV infection, an obligation founded not upon a prior agreement, nor upon any extraordinary moral obligations incumbent on health-care workers, but rather upon a consequentialist examination of the likely dangerous results if no such obligation is recognized. He adds that it is appropriate for Canadian society to begin consideration of a possible 'risk premium' tied to the occupational risk run by health workers caring for those who are HIV-infected.

H.A. Bassford provides a detailed examination of public health questions arising from screening for HIV infection: the use of 'quarantine' or isolation of those who are HIV-positive; the use of mandatory testing for certain population groups; the maintainance of confidentiality with respect to those who test positive for the HIV antibody; and the problems raised by HIV-positive persons who do not avoid high-risk activities. Using the principles that the moral purpose of civil society is to enable people to live well, and that any interferences in individual liberty should be as minimally restrictive as possible, Bassford argues against both the quarantine of infected persons and the mandatory screening of the general population or of so-called 'high-risk' populations, and defends education and voluntary screening as effective programs that both maintain individual autonomy and reduce the spread of infection.

Many PLWAs have forcefully protested against the difficulty of gaining access to non-validated drug treatments that might offer some possibility of relief of or improvement in their condition. Their interests in open access to possibly helpful drugs seem to conflict with the medical goal of scientific assessment of the effectiveness of drugs, an assessment that involves restriction of access and the use of double-blinded, randomized experiments, in which, of necessity, some subjects receive a placebo. In 'Catastrophic Rights: Vital Public Interests and Civil Liberties in Conflict', John Dixon assesses the merits of conservatism in drug regulation against the case for recognizing special rights of those with catastrophic illnesses such as AIDS. Dixon concludes that scientists must develop new ways of promoting controlled experimentation on catastrophic drugs while preserving, as far as possible, the therapeutic autonomy of the catastrophically ill PLWA.

As H.A. Bassford and B. Lee both point out, one important and essential approach to slowing the spread of HIV infection is the development of more and better education programs about AIDS, HIV, and the prevention of infection, directed towards the needs and interests of a variety of different audiences. Nevertheless, such educational materials are not value-free. In 'Warning: AIDS Health Promotion Programs May Be Hazardous to Your Autonomy', Patricia Illingworth raises some ethical questions about the content of certain materials used to educate 'the public' about AIDS. Insofar as these materials use manipulative techniques, she argues, they compromise the autonomy of those who are exposed to them, and further, in the absence of evidence that they are effective, they cannot be justified on the basis of a supposed promotion of the general welfare. Illingworth's discussion points in the direction of the development of accurate, effective education programs that enhance rather than compromise the self-determination of those for whom they are created.

Finally, it is important for Canadians to raise questions about appropriate health-care policies for those who have AIDS or are HIV-infected. In 'Living with AIDS: Toward Effective and Compassionate Health Care Policy', B. Lee documents the sorry Canadian history of 'state (in)action' in response to AIDS. Drawing upon the experiences of community AIDS groups, AIDS activists, and PLWAs themselves, he then outlines a comprehensive, sensitive, and practical set of policies for Canada, with suggestions about preventive programs to slow the spread of infection, and about appropriate forms of treatment, care, and support for people who are living with AIDS and HIV infection.

The crucial question for the whole of Canadian society is whether AIDS and HIV infection will continue to be constructed and interpreted in terms of a 'them' versus 'us' framework, or whether they can instead be dealt with from a perspective of mutual responsibility – responsibility for ourselves and for one another. In place of the sort of threatening and confounding approach to the epidemic exemplified by the billboard slogan, 'AIDS: Stick it in your head instead!', the papers in this volume show that Canadians can opt for careful reflection, moral sensitivity, and political awareness about AIDS and HIV infection.

NOTES

¹'AIDS Billboard Bungled in English Translation', *Kingston Whig-Standard* (26 June 1990), p. 3.

²Devon Worth, personal communication.

³Federal Centre for AIDS, 'Surveillance Update: AIDS in Canada' (Ottawa, 7 May 1990).

⁴See the excellent discussion of the concepts of promiscuity and the unnatural in Christine Pierce and Donald VanDeVeer, eds, *AIDS: Ethics and Public Policy* (Belmont, CA: Wadsworth, 1988), pp. 14-17.

⁵Robert Gallo, 'The AIDS Virus', *Scientific American* 256, 1 (January 1987): 46-56, and Peter Jaret, 'Our Immune System: The Wars Within', *National Geographic* 169, 6 (June 1986): 702-35.

⁶Federal Centre for AIDS, p. 2.

AIDS: THE SOCIAL DIMENSION

ARTHUR SCHAFER

INTRODUCTION

The AIDS epidemic may well become the greatest public health crisis of the twentieth century. There is widespread public recognition that it poses a fearful threat to the life and health of millions of people worldwide. There is also a recognition that the burden on our health-care system and on the national economy, already significant, is likely to increase dramatically. What is, perhaps, less widely appreciated is that our social responses to AIDS pose a serious threat to the shared attitudes and values that define us as a moral community.

If Canadians were invited to think about the total of accumulated capital in our society, most would likely take into account physical assets such as factories, mines, and office buildings, and the infra-structure of roads, railways, ports, and power grids. Only rarely would we think to include the complex of norms that makes possible and sustains all social activity. And yet these norms, which include respect for such values as rationality, altruism, public-spiritedness, and a sense of humanity, are no less essential to our social

1

survival and human flourishing than are the sources of power that drive the economic engine. Some would say that they are, if anything, more essential.[1]

Our social capital, not unlike our economic capital, can erode and dissipate if it is not properly maintained.[2] Perhaps we need to be reminded more frequently, by both cultural anthropologists and moral philosophers, that 'the normative order makes the factual order'.[3] That is, there exists in every society a fundamental set of cultural values that serves as a kind of social cement, binding individuals together into some kind of coherent community. At the same time, these foundational values define societies and give to each society its particular character.

Several of the basic values of Canadian society are threatened by our response(s) to the AIDS epidemic.

THE PLAGUE MENTALITY
Blaming the Victim

As Susan Sontag explains,[4] 'plague' is not simply a name for such frightening diseases as cholera, yellow fever, and typhoid. Derived from the Latin *plaga*, originally meaning stroke or wound, the word is now primarily used metaphorically. It signals a collective calamity, a great evil or scourge. In common parlance, not every epidemic qualifies as a plague, not even when the disease has a high mortality rate, as polio did and cancer does. It seems to be the case that in order to be counted as a plague, an epidemic must be conceptualized as possessing a moral dimension, something that is inflicted rather than merely endured, and that is deserved as a punishment for sin. As Father Paneloux comments, in Camus's novel *The Plague*:

> Calamity has come on you, my brethren, and you deserved it . . . the evil-doer has good cause to tremble. For plague is the flail of God and the world His threshing-floor, and implacably He will thresh out his harvest until the wheat is separated from the chaff.[5]

In every plague, the general population looks for some group to which blame can be attributed. The Black Death, for example, was blamed on the Jews, who were thought to have poisoned the wells (even though they themselves drank from the same wells as their fellow citizens).

Nor was the potentiality of plague to poison social relations confined to the distant past. The nineteenth-century European epidemics of Asiatic cholera were blamed by the rich on the poor, for being dirty and unhygienic. Indeed, the ruling classes in plague-stricken cities such as Hamburg came to regard the poor and vulnerable classes of society with almost complete contempt and fear, to the point of denying their human status. It may not be too far-fetched to link this insidious process of dehumanization to the subsequent popularity of Nazism in Hamburg, where the genocidal program of

2

sterilization and extermination proved more congenial than elsewhere in Germany.[6]

Although cholera was no respecter of social class, and drew its victims from the highest as well as the lowest strata of society, its inexorable spread was worst among those condemned to live in conditions of overcrowding, with no effective sewage disposal and insanitary waterways. Naturally enough, the poor predominated amongst its victims. It was obvious even at the time (e.g., to Dr Robert Koch, discoverer of the cholera bacillus) that the only sensible way of preventing 'the plague' was to improve living conditions for the poor, while introducing such measures as clean air and water. As Richard Evans demonstrates,[7] blaming the victims could only aggravate the public health crisis. Koch's sound advice was ignored until it was too late.

In every European country threatened by the nineteenth-century cholera epidemics, social conflicts and apprehensions were exacerbated. Whatever moral and political shortcomings existed in society were exposed mercilessly. British historian Asa Briggs makes the key point forcefully: the cholera plague was a 'profoundly social disease',[8] giving rise to rumours, suspicions, and conflicts. (Although mortality rates were even higher for tuberculosis, typhoid, smallpox, and measles, none of these diseases seems to have produced the psychological effect of cholera, which killed with alarming rapidity.)[9]

Epidemic diseases become prime candidates for plague status when the putative carriers of the epidemic are viewed as aliens, or marginal members of society, as 'the other' – because they are foreigners, or poor, or darker-skinned than the 'general population', or of the wrong religion, or the wrong sexual orientation.[10] Indeed, the very distinction, so easily and thoughtlessly accepted, between 'the general public', on the one hand, and risk groups, on the other, strongly reflects and reinforces the 'otherness' of those who are infected or infectious. Why do homosexuals not enjoy the same status – as charter members of the general public – that heterosexuals do? What begins as a seemingly inconsequential verbal point can unwittingly lead to increased willingness to support demands for their isolation or for their exclusion from ordinary legal rights and protections.

The AIDS epidemic fits most of the usual plague stereotypes, and well deserves the title 'God's gift to bigots'. It is believed to have originated in Africa, and to have spread from there to Haiti, North America, and then Europe. This hypothesis, whether or not it turns out ultimately to be correct, has great appeal to those who associate 'the dark continent' with sexual incontinence and primitive behaviour. In North America and Western Europe AIDS has spread most rapidly among the sub-culture of male homosexuals and intravenous drug users. An infectious disease whose primary means of transmission are 'deviant' sexual conduct and the use of illegal drugs is easily incorporated within the model of divine retribution for sin. The blame and opprobrium that are attached to both homosexuality and IV drug use (because of their association with sexual promiscuity and personal indulgence) produce in people who are not members of these 'risk groups' a feeling of moral smugness. The dangerous and deviant minorities are 'getting what they deserve'.

The tendency to identify some group(s) as scapegoats – the guilty ones who 'deserve' their fate but who threaten to spread their disease to the rest of us who are not deserving of such punishment – has, inevitably, a brutalizing effect upon society. It changes the hearts of men and women, weakening their human sympathies. It prevents many people from recognizing that the plague deeply concerns us all, not simply those stricken with the disease. In the words of Camus, describing the city of Oran after the onset of the plague, 'no longer were there individual destinies; only a collective destiny, made of plague and the emotions shared by all.'[11] It is a sad irony of history that the AIDS epidemic has occurred at just that time when, in Canadian society at least, homosexuality was beginning to gain acceptance as a statistical fact rather than as a moral blight. There is now a very real danger that the AIDS epidemic will produce a homophobic backlash.

The irrational propensity to search for some group(s) to scapegoat not only serves to undermine the sense we have of our common humanity, it also ensures that public health measures to contain 'the plague' cannot work effectively. In the case of AIDS, for example, if society stigmatizes and isolates those who have AIDS or who are seropositive for the HIV virus, there will be a strong disincentive to be tested for anyone who thinks that he or she may be at risk. The more punitive are society's attitudes towards those who test positive, the more will those individuals at risk avoid being tested. But if those 'at risk' refuse to be tested – going 'underground', if necessary – then society misses a vital opportunity to educate and counsel those who are infectious about the steps they should take to ensure that they do not infect others. There is thus a strong argument, based upon public health considerations, for avoiding strenuously the irrational temptation towards scapegoating and blaming the victim. Prudence and morality combine to support the same conclusion.

When the 'medical model' of disease is abandoned in favour of the 'moral model', there is a good likelihood that the results will be counter-productive and harmful in a variety of ways.

Xenophobia

We live in a world characterized by a high degree of international mobility. Interchange among people of different nationalities occurs in a number of different spheres: economic, cultural, and touristic. The xenophobia that typically characterizes the plague mentality often leads to hostility against immigrants and foreign visitors. This hostility may, in turn, result in the erection of barriers against foreign visitors. It may also promote intercommunal conflicts between 'the general community' and the community of immigrants.

In the Soviet Union, for example, news reports have stressed that foreigners are the prime source of HIV infection. This perception may well have influenced the Soviet government to adopt a policy requiring general testing (for HIV infectivity) of all foreigners who will be in the country for over three months, including students, tourists, and journalists. Those who refuse to take the test are subject to explusion.[12] The US Public Health Services has issued regulations requiring that immigrants be tested outside the country for infection with HIV, but this requirement does not apply to tourists, students, or resident foreign businessmen.

By contrast, there does not yet appear to be much public support in Canada for the efforts of a few demagogues to stir up feelings of xenophobia. It would, however, be naïve to suppose that there is no constituency for such dangerous over-reactions. If/when the level of public anxiety about AIDS rises sharply, a large constituency for such policies could easily develop. In every society, including Canada, there is a reservoir of distrust, suspicion, and ignorance that offers a fertile breeding ground for public hostility. In order to diminish the danger of such over-reaction, public health officials will be required repeatedly to stress the fact that the unavoidable interconnectedness of the modern world renders all such isolationist efforts futile. This prudential appeal could be buttressed by a moral appeal focusing upon the common humanity shared by citizens of every nation. The image of country after country isolating itself and its people behind a series of new 'Berlin Walls' is as ugly as it is ludicrous.

Certainly, very few thoughtful Canadians are likely to support proposals that we should seal our borders tightly against all foreigners – not once they appreciate that this would mean forgoing the economic benefits of tourism, foreign trade, and international business, not to mention the hardship that this would impose upon separated families and friends. But there is a worrying possibility that certain ethnic and racial minorities within Canada – such as Africans or Caribbeans – could face increased prejudice and discrimination. The media are already suggesting that sex with 'people from overseas' is a risky behaviour. 'People from overseas' is a thinly veiled code phrase for Africans and Caribbeans. The view is subtly reinforced that if 'we' avoid intimate relations with 'them', we can avoid AIDS.[13]

As a more effective and humane alternative to the punitive approach to epidemic disease, one might hope that the policy of the Canadian government would be supportive of efforts towards increased international cooperation, in the field of medical research and also in other measures necessary to promote global public health.

Irrationality

Of all the values threatened by the plague mentality, critical rationality is in some ways the most important and the most vulnerable.

Rationality is, almost invariably, the first casualty of any 'plague'. Fear of the unknown and inability to tolerate uncertainty tend to generate what might be called 'apocalyptic thinking'. In modern Canada, no less than medieval Europe, many people opt for the simplistic explanations that are confidently propounded by demagogues in preference to the complex hypotheses that are tentatively advanced by epidemiologists and scientific researchers. Since scientific explanations must frequently be adjusted or abandoned when they run afoul of inconvenient facts, they can never achieve the certitude of pseudo-moralistic explanations, whose very invulnerability to refutation is what disqualifies them from the status of genuine science.

It is worth noting that even in the superstitious world of fourteenth-century Europe, there was a minority, including some public health officials, who recognized the connection between environmental factors, such as rats, and the bubonic plague. As a result, there were some limited attempts at rat control. For most people, though, it was simply easier and more attractive to blame the plague on Anointers and Jews. Bigotry, superstition, and ignorance had an easy win over scientific rationality.

When one reads that suburban communities around Toronto declined to participate in that city's public-health program to combat AIDS (at the cost of a few dollars per resident) on the grounds that AIDS was largely an inner-city problem, one cannot help feeling a certain *déjà vu*. The irrational tendency to treat epidemic disease as 'someone else's problem' persists even when the disease reservoir is at the city gates, as it were.

Since not everyone recognizes that rationality is among the core values of Western culture, it is important that we remind ourselves just why any threat to the value of rationality represents, at the same time, a serious threat to the very survival of our culture.

The struggle of our species to win a living from nature has been a long and difficult one. Even now, only a small part of the world's population enjoys any sort of material comfort. Most are condemned to an existence marked by poverty and disease. Whatever doubts one may have about the science and technology of Western civilization, it is beyond argument that such progress as we have achieved has depended in an important way upon the development of critical thinking: the habit of mind that honestly and patiently collects evidence with which to test our beliefs. Progress in agriculture, transportation, communications, and health could have come about in no other way. If we have, to some limited extent, managed to transcend the ignorance and poverty of our forebears, it is because, in our culture, blind superstition has partly given way to a more rigorous ethics of belief. The ethos of critical rationality insists that we apportion the confidence we place in our beliefs to the evidence available. When there is good evidence against a proposition, it should be disbelieved. When there is no good evidence for or against a proposition, we ought to suspend belief.

Perhaps no philosopher has given a more eloquent defence of the importance of strict rationality in our belief system than the nineteenth-century

British writer William Kingdon Clifford. Clifford's ethics of belief is nicely summarized in his declaration that 'it is wrong always, everywhere and for any one, to believe anything upon insufficient evidence'. Clifford argues that no real belief, however trifling it may seem, is ever truly insignificant, for

> it prepares us to receive more of its like, confirms those which resembled it before, and weakens others; and so gradually it lays a stealthy train in our inmost thoughts, which may someday explode into overt action, and leave its stamp upon our character forever.[14]

Although the adoption of a smugly moralistic tone towards the sufferers from an epidemic, such as AIDS, may give pleasure to some people, the pleasure is epistemically 'stolen' and therefore morally condemnable. No one is entitled to believe that AIDS represents divine punishment for sin when the distribution of the disease is such that many 'sinners' go unpunished and many 'non-sinners' become ill and die. As an aside, one might marvel at the elaborate mental contortions that enable religious fundamentalists to explain away the fact that lesbians are the group least at risk for AIDS infection. Is there, perhaps, some as yet undiscovered divine significance in this phenomenon?

Our beliefs and our modes of thinking are not simply private matters. They are common property, an inheritance to be passed on to succeeding generations. We have no more stringent duty than to guard the rationality of our beliefs by ensuring that they are based upon adequate evidence. Belief that is given indiscriminately degrades the believers and endangers their fellows. Belief that is based upon carefully tested evidence, after fair and full enquiry, binds people together and strengthens the human community.[15]

In the context of Canadian responses to AIDS, it may be useful to consider some illustrative examples of irrational thinking, together with its demonstrably harmful consequences.

North American physicians have known for some time that the HIV virus is not casually transmissible. To mention just one of many recent studies, it has been reported in *The New England Journal of Medicine* that 'of the more than 30,000 cases of AIDS in the United States reported to the Centers for Disease Control by February 1987, none have [*sic*] occurred in family members of patients with AIDS, unless the members have had other recognized risk-related behaviour.'[16] Although the majority of household contacts shared household facilities, including beds, toilets, bathing facilities, and kitchens, as well as items likely to be soiled by patients' saliva or body fluids (e.g., eating utensils, plates, drinking glasses, and towels), none of the studies could demonstrate even a single HIV infection among household members who did not have additional exposure to HIV infection through blood, sexual activity, or perinatal transmission.

Despite all this evidence, some physicians and nurses persist in masking and gloving up in order simply to converse with AIDS patients by their bedside.

When challenged, these health-care workers sometimes acknowledge that their behaviour is irrational, but justify themselves with the claim that donning mask and gloves makes them feel psychologically more comfortable.

When one considers the wider implications of such behaviour, however, it may be seen as very damaging from a number of points of view. First, it represents an indignity towards patients with AIDS, further isolating and stigmatizing them. More than this, however, it sends an entirely inappropriate and dangerous message to the public. At the same time as community health officials offer reassurance to the public that there is no need to quarantine persons with AIDS, and no danger to anyone who works or studies alongside persons with AIDS, some physicians are signalling, by their behaviour, that they believe the HIV virus to be casually transmissible. The inconsistent behaviour of physicians (or other health-care workers) who 'say one thing and do another' illustrates how irrationality is not merely a personal foible to be indulged but an impermissible violation of the ethical injunction to do no harm.

Consider: a seventy-eight-year-old woman was recently refused admission by four different Nova Scotia nursing homes because she carried the AIDS virus. She had contracted the virus from a transfusion of contaminated blood during an operation in 1985. Although she had not shown symptoms of the disease and her immune system was stable, she required care in a nursing home because she was suffering from severe arthritis.

Consider: Reverend Charles Farnsworth, headmaster of the Grenville Christian School, in Brockville, Ontario, where a mandatory AIDS-testing policy has recently been introduced, declared that a positive AIDS test would lead to exclusion from the privately run school. He acknowledged that much of the fear about AIDS transmission may be rooted in ignorance, but insisted that 'people's fears must be respected'.

Consider: Volunteer firemen refused to respond to a call for help from a Roman Catholic monastery that cares for babies with AIDS. Two firemen from the nearby Annapolis Volunteer Fire Brigade refused to answer an emergency call for oxygen when one of the babies began choking. The infant died several days later.

Consider: In a survey carried out during the summer of 1988, it was revealed that 56 per cent of 1,500 Canadians surveyed believed that working alongside a fellow employee with AIDS would constitute a workplace hazard. They favoured compulsory testing of all prospective employees. Similar testing was not favoured for drug or alcohol addiction, despite a barrage of negative publicity about its harmful effects in the workplace.

Consider: The St James-Assiniboia School Division in Winnipeg has assured parents that it is safe to allow teachers or pupils with AIDS to continue in school, but it has spent thousands of dollars purchasing rubber gloves for teachers in case a child should have a bleeding nose or be cut in a playground accident.

Consider: Large numbers of Canadian medical-school students are strongly advocating compulsory AIDS testing for all hospital patients. When reminded that a negative test is no guarantee that the patient is not infectious, and that hospital policy recommends that full precautions be taken during every risky medical procedure, students continue to insist adamantly upon the need for compulsory testing. Whatever may be the adverse consequences for patients, these students 'want to know'. Moreover, many declare that if they were to learn that a patient was HIV-positive, they would refuse treatment. Some would plan their internship and residency training so as to avoid institutions in high-risk areas. Their attitude does not change significantly when informed of the epidemiological data showing no greater risk of AIDS among health-care workers than among the rest of the population.

Each of these Canadian examples illustrates dramatically William Clifford's thesis that irrationality in seemingly insignificant matters can produce, directly or indirectly, gravely harmful consequences for one's fellow human beings. If the medical community is going to tell parents that it is safe to send their children to school alongside a schoolmate or teacher who is HIV-positive, and if they are going to tell workers that it is safe to work alongside a colleague who is HIV-positive, and if they are going to tell the public that it is safe to eat in restaurants where a chef or waiter is HIV-positive, then it will not do for doctors to behave as if they really believe that AIDS is casually transmissible. It may not be possible for any of us entirely to eradicate all irrational fears about AIDS transmission. It should be possible for all of us to resist acting on the basis of such fears.

De-socialization

Canadian society is often described by cultural commentators as 'individualistic'. Although this term is not used with precision, it is usually meant to suggest a constellation of values that includes emphasis on individual rights and liberties, self-fulfillment, privacy, independence, and personal autonomy.[17] Individualism, in this sense, is a central norm of Canadian society. But whereas individualism is only one of the central norms of Canadian society, it is *the* defining ideal of American society.

American culture proudly affirms the worth of the single individual, unconstrained in body or in mind, entirely independent of his fellows.[18] Much of American literature celebrates the worth of the totally liberated, atomistic individual (as in the writings of Emerson and Thoreau). Critics of American culture such as Daniel Callahan[19] and Christopher Lasch[20] are concerned that an excessive preoccupation with self, at the expense of community, has led America into a 'tyranny of individualism' so great as to threaten that nation's cultural survival.

The sharp antinomy between the individual and the state, so often observed in American culture, is much softened in Canadian culture by the stress on such mediating group loyalties as regionalism (we are not simply

Canadians, we are Maritimers or Westerners or Québécois) and ethnicity. Although it has become a cliché, our symbol of 'the cultural mosaic', by contrast with the American symbol of 'the melting pot', points to the existence of strong popular identification with sub-cultures and sub-communities of various sorts. Moreover, again in contradistinction to our southern neighbours, Canadians have been historically altogether more enthusiastic about the interventionist role of governments at all levels. The government is expected to speak powerfully on behalf of the interests of the broader community, for example, by using taxing powers to fund such community programs as medicare and public education.

There is reason to fear that what we are calling 'the plague mentality' could so affect the tenor of Canadian social life that we too could follow the Americans into a state of hyper-individualism. The present balance between the pursuit of self-interest, on the one hand, and public-spiritedness, on the other, could descend into the unbridled pursuit of self-interest. The danger is that our society could come more closely to resemble Hobbes's 'state of nature', in which the life of man was 'solitary, poor, nasty, brutish and short'. The process of de-socialization has already begun, and unless we are vigilant, it could accelerate.

Every society functions on a symbolical no less than on a practical level. The political life of a community is heavily dependent upon its symbolic life.[21] Fear and suspicion of other people, any one of whom is potentially a carrier of the murderous HIV virus, could seriously erode our already frail bonds of compassion and trust. As Daniel Callahan explains, in hard times options are fewer, choices nastier. Blaming and denunciation become more congenial than forgiveness and therapy. If life is going poorly, someone obviously must be at fault. The warm, expansive self gives way to the harsh, competitive self; enemies abound, foreign and domestic. Incivility or even nastiness become the norm.[22] The problem is, of course, that it is precisely during 'hard times' that a society most needs to invoke the values of altruism, public-spiritedness, and civility.

Camus perceptively describes the inevitable tension between the need for human solidarity and the fear of contagion created by the plague mentality:

> people, . . . though they have an instinctive craving for human contacts, can't bring themselves to yield to it, because of the mistrust that keeps them apart. For it's common knowledge that you can't trust your neighbour; he may pass the disease to you without your knowing it, and take advantage of a moment of inadvertence on your part to infect you.[23]

Once avoidance and exclusion become the norm, we have lost a vital community resource. The plague 'within each of us' is not the submicroscopic virus as much as it is an extreme alienation from our fellow human beings. Canada could become, if we are not careful, the kind of society in which passersby ignore the needs of accident victims, for fear of contamination through contact with blood, a society in which even the most chaste and faithful harbour a dread of other people.

Some may find this an unduly pessimistic scenario; but there is considerable evidence from social scientists in support of the view that socially co-operative behaviour does decrease when bonds of trust are attenuated by negative feelings. For example, the psychologist Harvey Hornstein and his colleagues discovered,[24] in the midst of their 'wallet-returning' experiment, that on 4 June 1968, the day Robert F. Kennedy was murdered, not one of the wallets that they set out was returned. Since the rate of return prior to this event had been a fairly steady 40 per cent, one is led to infer that people's feelings about the moral community in which they live can have a significant influence on their behaviour. When people develop negative feelings about their fellows, they become less public-spirited.

More than a century ago, Alexis De Tocqueville observed, in *Democracy in America*, that unbridled competitive individualism was leading towards a dangerous social fragmentation. There is today, in the era of AIDS, a great relevance to his warnings against a social environment in which man is 'ceaselessly throw[n] back on himself, alone, and confined entirely in the solitude of his own heart'. In our understandable concern for the looming public health crisis, we must not overlook the concomitant threat to community values. Spiritual impoverishment could prove to be one of the worst consequences of the AIDS epidemic. To counteract this possibility should be among our highest priorities.

CONCLUSION

The conclusion to which the arguments of this chapter point is that the AIDS epidemic is as much a threat to our cultural values as it is to our lives, our health-care system, and our economy. The phrase 'plague mentality' encapsulates a series of attitudes and values: victim blaming, xenophobia, irrationality, and de-socialization. There is still time to counteract, decisively, the plague mentality. The survival of our common humanity is at stake.

NOTES

[1]Fred Hirsch, *The Social Limits of Growth* (London: Routledge and Kegan Paul, 1977).

[2]James Coleman, 'Norms as Social Capital'. In Gerard Radnitzky and Peter Bernholtz, eds, *Economic Imperialism* (New York: Paragon House, 1986).

[3]Kingsley Davis, *Human Society* (New York: Macmillan, 1949), p. 53.

[4]Susan Sontag, *AIDS And Its Metaphors* (London: Allen Lane/Penguin Press, 1989), p. 44.

[5]Albert Camus, *The Plague* (London: Penguin Books, 1960), p. 80.

[6]Richard J. Evans, *Death in Hamburg: Society and Politics in the Cholera Years 1830-1910* (Oxford: Oxford University Press, 1988).

[7]Ibid.

[8]Asa Briggs, 'Cholera and Society in the Nineteenth Century'. *Past and Present* 19 (April 1961).

[9]William H. McNeill, *Plagues and Peoples* (New York: Anchor/Doubleday, 1967).

[10]Sontag, *AIDS And Its Metaphors*.

[11]Camus, *The Plague*, p. 138.

[12]Unsigned news note, *Hastings Centre Report*, 'Foreigners and Fears', December 1987, p.3

[13]Rachel Murray, 'Worlds Apart'. *The New Statesman and Society*, 6 October 1989, p. 20.

[14]William Kingdon Clifford, *The Scientific Basis of Morals* (New York: J. Fitzgerald, 1884), p. 26.

[15]Ibid.

[16]H. Friedland and R.H.S. Klein, 'Transmission of the Human Immunodeficiency Virus'. *New England Journal of Medicine* 317, no. 18 (29 October 1987), p. 1132.

[17]For a fuller discussion of the concept of individualism, see, e.g., Stephen Lukes, *Individualism* (New York: Harper and Row, 1973); and Christopher Lasch, 'Birth, Death and Technology: The Limits of Cultural Laissez-faire', *Hastings Centre Review* 2 (June 1972).

[18]See, e.g., John William Ward, 'Individualism: Ideology or Utopia?', *Hastings Centre Studies* 2, no. 3 (Sept. 1974); and Daniel Callahan, *The Tyranny of Survival* (New York: Macmillan, 1973), chap. 5, 'The Tyranny of Individualism'.

[19]Callahan, *The Tyranny of Survival*.

[20]Lasch, 'Birth, Death and Technology'.

[21]Michael Novak, 'The Social World of Individuals', *Hastings Centre Studies* 2, no. 3 (Sept. 1974).

[22]Callahan, 'Minimalist Ethics: On the Pacification of Morality'. In Arthur L. Caplan and Daniel Callahan, *Ethics In Hard Times* (New York: Plenum Press, 1981), pp. 261-2.

[23]Camus, *The Plague*, p. 160.

[24]Harvey Hornstein, Elisha Fisch, and Michael Holmes. 'Influence of a Model's Feelings About His Behaviour and His Relevance as a Comparison Other on Observers' Helping Behaviour', *Journal of Personality and Social Psychology* 10 (1968), pp. 220-6.

AIDS AND DISABILITY

––––––––

JEROME E. BICKENBACH

In North America, the social perception of AIDS has been almost entirely formed by the fact that it is a sexually transmitted disease, the greatest burden of which has been borne by the gay community. Though it is common knowledge that there are non-sexual modes of transmission, and victims of the disease other than homosexual males, the perception persists, and is daily reinforced by the media, that the AIDS epidemic raises, above all, questions of sexual morality.[1]

As a general matter, the social perception of a contagious disease – and the metaphors that shape our public discourse about it[2] – will profoundly affect the debate over the kinds of social measures required to alter its course. In a society such as ours, committed by law and liberal political tradition to the protection of both individual rights and general welfare, this important debate must resolve tensions between equally important but conflicting interests. In particular, our social response to an epidemic must weigh the rights of those already infected against the rights of those who are not, and must balance the effectiveness of public health measures in checking the epidemic against the sacrifices those measures demand of individual citizens.

In the case of the AIDS epidemic, the sexual dimension of the disease has undoubtedly distorted this debate. Attitudes about sexuality have hampered the planning and implementation of 'safe sex' campaigns, even though they are by far the least intrusive of the traditional repertoire of public health measures. Health officials have had to contend not only with delicate sensibilities, but also with the widely held belief that by encouraging the use of condoms, they are condoning promiscuity. Far more damaging, though, has been the belief that AIDS is the result of a blameworthy failure of sexual self-restraint, a moral lapse that calls forth its own punishment.

There has been, in short, a partial fusion of issues of health policy and the politics of sexual orientation. As we struggle to confront the epidemic, the distortions of the sexual dimension will continue to prejudice the interests of the AIDS victim, aligned with socially vulnerable, 'high-risk' populations and stigmatized by a vague but powerful image of sexual impropriety.

Should politicians and public health officials try to alter the social perception of AIDS by de-emphasizing its association with sexual morality? It is not clear how successful this would be, or if it would be worth the massive cost of public re-education. It would be far more sensible to revise existing frameworks for social-policy development, since these are more flexible and can be explicitly altered by legislation, enforceable regulations, and ministerial policy guidelines. The question then becomes, what aspects of the disease should be emphasized?

Ironically, the most obvious dimension of AIDS has received the least attention: AIDS is a disease syndrome, brought about by viral infection, that, because it impairs organic functions, acts to restrict or limit normal human activities. In other words, AIDS qualifies as a *physical disability*, as defined by the World Health Organization.[3] Moreover, this is an intrinsic feature of AIDS, since if it had no disabling consequences, AIDS would, quite properly, be ignored by public health officials. In contrast, though foremost in the public's mind, the connection between AIDS and sexual conduct is not intrinsic – it is nothing more than an epidemiological accident. Clearly AIDS would pose a serious threat to public health even if no one contracted it sexually, and none of those infected were homosexual.

But AIDS is more than a physical disability; it is also a *physical handicap*. Although we ordinarily treat these two terms as synonyms, there is an implicit conceptual difference between them that should be highlighted. This is the difference between having a disabling physical condition and being socially disadvantaged because of it. We should emphasize this difference for the simple reason that not every disability has adverse social consequences, like stigmatization and discrimination. Some people with disabilities are handicapped, others are not. Thus the World Health Organization has defined a physical handicap as 'a disadvantage for a given individual, resulting from an impairment or a disability, that limits or pre-vents the fulfilment of a role that is normal . . . for that individual.' In this respect, AIDS certainly seems to qualify as a handicap.

What are the advantages of emphasizing this dimension of the disease? This is not an idle question, since, from the perspective of a person with AIDS, it may seem that all that is involved here is a shift from one form of stigmati-zation to another. Although people with physical disabilities are rarely per-ceived as sexual deviants, they often face denial of equal access to services and opportunities, assumptions of inferiority and failure, and paternalistic treat-ment that undermines autonomy and self-respect. To make matters worse, those whose disabilities are viewed as self-inflicted – which is often how AIDS is perceived – may have to bear the additional burden of moral blame or sanctimonious aversion.

There is no doubt that handicapped people face these and other forms of oppression in our culture. But the fact remains that people with AIDS bear most of this burden already, and could only benefit from a closer affiliation with people with disabilities. For the two groups have much in common: both regularly confront discrimination in employment, public accommoda-tion, and education. Both must contend with institutionalization, quarantin-ing, guardianship, and other restrictions on their liberty. And both share the frustrations involved in obtaining information about, and input into, medical research. If nothing else, by joining in the cause of people with disabilities, people with AIDS would lose their isolation – a precondition to the long-range goal of increased self-empowerment.[4]

Furthermore, from the wider perspective of policy formation on AIDS issues, the shift from the domain of sexual morality to that of entitlements for people with disabilities is potentially very useful. In the absence of clearly articulated policy, it is inevitable that courts of law and human-rights tribu-nals will be called upon to resolve specific disputes raised by the AIDS epidemic. The law with respect to the rights of people with disabilities has already evolved legal principles and tests for dealing with similar disputes, and this legal framework can help to clarify the larger social debate involving AIDS.

In short, the laws of Canada and the United States already offer some valuable tools for making a start at resolving both of the tensions created by the AIDS epidemic – that of weighing the rights of those infected against the rights of those who are not, and that of balancing the effectiveness of public health measures against the sacrifices they entail. In this instance, public health officials can learn a great deal from legal theory.

AIDS AS DISABILITY AND HANDICAP

But before we turn to the legal principles, are there any conceptual difficulties in treating AIDS as a disability and a handicap? Two related problems come to mind. First, unlike other physical disabilities, such as blindness, deafness, epilepsy, and cerebral palsy, AIDS is a contagious disease. Second, it is not entirely clear what it means to 'have AIDS'. That is, because AIDS is a complex medical syndrome, involving a spectrum of opportunistic and infectious diseases, there are various categories of AIDS victims.[5] Besides those with full-blown AIDS, there are others who have tested HIV-seropositive but are otherwise asymptomatic; still others have a milder form of immunodeficiency called AIDS-Related Complex, or ARC.

The first objection is easily dealt with: clearly, the fact that people with AIDS can transmit the disease in no way argues against their being physically disabled. Contagiousness is simply a feature that certain disabling conditions possess, a feature that happens to bring about the same disabling condition in others.

But then, could it be argued that when people with AIDS are discriminated against in accommodation or employment, the basis for this treatment is not their disabling condition, as such, but their contagiousness? This is just to make the mistake of trying to detach one intrinsic feature of a disability from others.[6] Still, there is a genuine concern here that takes us to the second, more substantial, objection to considering AIDS not merely as a disability, but also as a handicap.

It might be argued that the contagiousness of asymptomatic HIV carriers is not directly linked to a physical disability they actually have; indeed, some projections suggest that there is a fairly good chance they will never develop the disease. Though HIV antibodies can be found in their bloodstream, and they can infect others, it would be very tempting to say that these people are healthy. Does this mean they are neither disabled nor handicapped?

The point is worth making, first off, that we do not know enough about HIV infection to be able to say with any confidence that someone can be a carrier of the virus and yet 'healthy'. It may well be, for example, that everyone infected sooner or later develops some form of immune-system deficiency. But as well, and more to the point, what limits an asymptomatic HIV carrier is not merely the physical condition of HIV-seropositivity. In addition, and necessarily, the various consequences and social ramifications of that condition impose restrictions. In this case, then, 'disability' is both a physical and social, or normative, phenomenon. Carriers are not disfunctional in any straightforward biological sense; they can, physically, engage in unprotected sex, become pregnant, or donate sperm. It is a different matter, though true enough, that they have a moral duty and a legal obligation not to do these things.

This is a fair point, but not particularly decisive. For, to one degree or another, all physical disabilities have this dual feature. In nearly all cases the physical condition itself (being blind, or deaf, or hypoglycaemic) restricts normal activities in part by virtue of the projects and goals the person has, or is socially expected to have.[7] Admittedly, all of the commonly recognized physical disabilities also limit some aspect of basic, physiological function-ing, wholly independently of social expectations or personal goals. And that is a difference, since an HIV carrier might conceivably live out a normal lifespan without experiencing any physiological disfunctioning. But is that enough to settle the question whether the carrier has a disability or not?

It could be that the notion of disability, even as defined by the World Health Organization, is simply not precise enough definitely to include or exclude the case of the asymptomatic HIV carrier. If so, from the perspective of policy formation, we should at least ensure that we have good reasons for including or excluding asymptomatic carriers from this category, and take care not to confuse this decision with other important social decisions, such as whether we should restrict where they can work or with whom they can associate.

It may also be the case that the real worry here does not directly concern the concept of disability at all. For whether or not it qualifies as a disability, being an asymptomatic HIV carrier will certainly be socially disadvantageous in a variety of ways. That is, the carrier may be handicapped even if she or he is not disabled.

Here some recent law may be able to help. A lawyer would approach this question by considering the rationale for having a legal category of people with handicaps, and then asking if the social decision to include or exclude asymptomatic HIV carriers would comport with that rationale. Following this line of reasoning, the result is clear enough. Since we have the legal category in part to prevent, or at least remedy, discrimination against people because of bias, ignorance, and other misperceptions that are associated with a physical condition, and since discrimination of this sort is easily imagined in the case of asymptomatic HIV carriers, they should be deemed to be handicapped.[8]

As far as the law is concerned, in other words, it is more important to provide a remedy for an evil – discrimination on the basis of disability – than to come up with a medically or philosophically acceptable characterization of the antecedents of handicaps. Thus the legal definition of 'physical handi-cap' in Canada and United States is very wide; so wide, indeed, as to include not only asymptomatic HIV carriers, but also anyone who is perceived – even incorrectly – to be physically or mentally disabled. And, following similar reasoning, in 1988 the Canadian Human Rights Commission extended its protection to cover individuals who belong to high-risk groups (whether they have AIDS or not), or associate with people with AIDS or members of high risk-groups.[9] In law, then, even perfectly healthy people can be handi-capped.

However conceptually odd such a 'definition' might appear, the back-ground rationale is morally sound: as a society we sometimes make special provisions for groups of people identified by some characteristic that has made them vulnerable to stigmatization and discriminatory treatment.

Questions about how that characteristic is to be precisely defined, or whether someone discriminated against actually possesses that characteristic, are relatively trivial concerns compared with the genuine problem of deciding what is to be done to remedy the situation.

In short, the fact that AIDS is a contagious disease and that some carriers are otherwise asymptomatic is irrelevant to the claim that people with AIDS, of whatever category, are physically handicapped in the World Health Organization sense. 'Handicap' is not a medical notion at all; it is a sociological or political one. That said, though, it must also be emphasized that relevant medical information about the disease may make all the difference in how we approach the conflicts and dilemmas the AIDS epidemic has brought about.

'SUFFICIENT RISK' AND 'REASONABLE ACCOMMODATION'

The Federal Centre for AIDS in Ottawa estimates that up to 50,000 Canadians may be HIV-positive. Of these only a very few are immobile or require hospitalization; most people with AIDS are physically able to carry on with their lives. Since they are contagious, however, the question arises whether it is fair to expose others to the risk of infection.

One context in which this issue has been repeatedly raised is the workplace.[10] Here the tension between equally legitimate interests is often dramatic. Persons with AIDS call for equal treatment and the right to carry on with jobs they are qualified and fit to perform. Their co-workers, however, insist that they have a right to a safe and healthy working environment, a concern also shared by customers and clients. How might such disputes be fairly resolved?

Suppose that a qualified primary-school teacher who is HIV-infected, but otherwise healthy, is fired from a teaching job because of fear of contagion – a fear voiced by both co-workers and parents. The teacher brings an action under one of the provincial Human Rights Codes, charging discrimination on the basis of physical handicap.[11] To what legal principles and analyses would a provincial human-rights tribunal turn in order to adjudicate this complaint?

Given the very broad legal definition, the tribunal would have no trouble finding that the teacher was physically handicapped. Nor could there be much dispute that the teacher had been fired because of that handicap. Thus the onus would immediately shift to the school board, as employer, to justify its actions. In particular, the school board would be called upon to persuade the tribunal that in the circumstances, and taking into consideration the interests of all people involved, outright dismissal was the only appropriate course of action open to it.

The school board would undoubtedly begin by pointing to its legal duty to provide a safe workplace, a duty arising from occupational health and safety legislation, collective agreements, and ministerial policy. It would then argue that the dismissal was justified inasmuch as the nature and extent of the disability made the teacher 'incapable of performing or fulfilling the essential duties or requirements' of the job.[12] In effect, that is, the employer would argue that being free of HIV infection is a bona fide, reasonable, and legitimate precondition to employment as a teacher. Insisting that this precondition be met, the board would conclude, is the only feasible way of satisfying their legal duties and protecting all the interests involved.

In adjudicating this claim, the tribunal would rely on a two-stage analysis. It would first ask whether the continued presence of the teacher on the job would pose a 'sufficient risk' to the health and safety of others. To make this judgement it would ask for evidence of the nature, duration, and severity of the risk, and, in particular, the likelihood of transmission in the school environment. Public perceptions of the risk, or commonly held but unsupportable fears about modes of transmission, are of no interest to the tribunal; it seeks medical information. As well, what is required is medical evidence with respect to the risk actually posed by *this* teacher in *this* working environment.

Given what we now know about the modes of transmission of the AIDS virus, the risk of HIV infection from a teacher in the school environment is so minimal as to count, at best, as a theoretical possibility.[13] A theoretical risk, however, is not a 'sufficient risk'. It is not 'sufficient' because the point of the legal standard is to identify a non-minimal level of risk, a risk that, as a society, we will accept as reasonable when competing interests are at stake. Thus the chances are quite good that the school board would be unable to show that the teacher was, by virtue of HIV positivity, unqualified to hold the job. As a result, dismissal being neither appropriate nor necessary, the school board would be asked to reinstate the teacher.

Suppose, though, that instead of being a teacher, the complainant was a medical technician regularly exposed to transfusable blood, or an emergency-room nurse, or an osteopathic surgeon. In these cases, the likelihood of transmission is significantly increased and the risk of infection no longer 'theoretical'. In these employment circumstances, a human-rights tribunal might well be convinced that the risk was sufficient to warrant dismissal. If it does, however, that is not the end of the matter. It must now be asked why dismissal was the only feasible course of action open to the employer.

In this second stage of the analysis, the tribunal asks whether 'reasonable accommodation' would enable the HIV-infected employee to continue working without exposing others to unacceptable levels of risk. What is reasonable accommodation? In the employment context, 'accommodation' normally involves job restructuring or reassignment, the acquisition of new equipment and special aids, or the adoption or modification of appropriate procedures and protocols.[14] And accommodation is reasonable, according to the current legal test, if it would not unduly burden the employer.

In order to make the argument that she or he will be burdened unduly, the employer would undoubtedly raise considerations of cost, technical feasibility, the requirements imposed by health and safety regulations, inconvenience, and similar considerations. The tribunal's job will then be to look at this evidence, assess it, and reach a judgement. Should it decide that reasonable means for accommodating the HIV-infected employee do exist, then it may order that these be put into place. Otherwise, the employee with AIDS will have to look for other employment.

Of course, the law in this area is far less clear and settled than this somewhat idealized outline suggests. Still, we can detach the 'sufficient risk'/'reasonable accommodation' analysis from its legal moorings and independently assess it as a model for public-health policy – as a method, that is, for setting out, and resolving, conflicts of interests created by the AIDS epidemic. And viewed as a general framework for making decisions about health measures, the analysis certainly has valuable features to recommend it.

First of all, the analysis is easily applicable to other AIDS-related conflicts. It would be appropriate, for example, to apply both the sufficient risk and the reasonable accommodation tests to the dilemma of whether to allow HIV-infected children to continue in the normal school program. The same analysis could also be used to resolve the conflict between a person with AIDS needing medical, dental, or psychiatric care and a health-care worker who, fearing infection, refused to provide that care. It might also help to settle disputes between people with AIDS and their landlords.

In addition, the 'sufficient risk'/'reasonable accommodation' analysis places most of the onus of proof on those who would limit the rights of people with AIDS. This is essential because, in the society at large, people with AIDS constitute (and, one hopes, will continue to constitute) a very small minority whose voice can easily be drowned out by the demands of an apprehensive majority. The analysis also requires a realistic and scientifically accurate determination of risk of infection, an important safeguard against the distortive effects of misinformation and misperception. As well, the analysis insists upon a case-by-case determination of both the risks to others and the ways of accommodating those who are HIV-infected, the two most salient aspects of conflicts between those who have a contagious disease and those who do not.

Finally, the analysis is founded, implicitly, on the premiss that people with physical disabilities must be treated as equals, with a right to equal participation in all facets of society. Because of this focus, the issue of sexual morality need never be raised when the analysis is applied to AIDS. Instead, HIV infection can be viewed as a physical handicap that results from a life-threatening, as yet incurable, and contagious disease syndrome. The analysis proceeds on the assumption that risks to others can be realistically assessed, and, in the usual instance, accommodated without imposing an undue burden on the healthy, or resorting to the drastic measure of preventing people with AIDS from engaging in the normal social activities of living.

Despite all these virtues, there is a popular objection to this or any other policy model that seeks to balance interests. We have only two options, the objector will insist. Either we try to secure the greatest health benefit for all, and ignore considerations of rights or equality, or else we accept the cost in public health that protection of rights and equality might entail. Though we may be tempted by the second, only the first option is socially acceptable, for the simple reason that we can never be certain of the actual health risks posed by an epidemic. When the stakes are as high as they are in the case of AIDS (the argument goes) we cannot afford our cherished political values; short of medical certainty, as a matter of policy, we should always err on the side of caution and put considerations of rights or equality in abeyance.

In effect, this objection suggests that our standard for 'sufficient risk' should be set as low as possible, so that the merest possibility of a risk is sufficient to justify unequal and right-infringing treatment. But the point of the objection is quite general and applies to any public-health measure thought to be of assistance in dealing with AIDS. Compulsory testing and reporting, involuntary contact tracing, forced quarantining of non-compliant HIV carriers, criminal restrictions on forms of sexual conduct: these and other intrusive measures could easily be justified as having potential – which is say, merely possible – epidemiological benefits.

This objection leads us to the second tension created by the AIDS epidemic, that of balancing the effectiveness of public-health measures against the sacrifices those measures require of everyone, healthy and ill alike. How can the law's approach to the rights and interests of people with disabilities assist us here?

'PROPER PURPOSE' AND 'REASONABLE LIMITS'

In Canada there is no doubt that the federal legislature has the constitutional authority to enact emergency health measures of the sort needed to confront an epidemic.[15] But what are the limits of that authority? Historically, English and Canadian courts were reluctant to question the rationale or necessity of public-health measures. Yet even early on, when courts were far more deferential to Parliament than they are now, it was never thought that this authority was unlimited. When a court dismissed the claim that an individual's privacy or right to property was infringed by quarantining or compulsory vaccination, it was in effect saying that these personal sacrifices do not undermine the legitimacy of the state's authority to deal with a public-health emergency. In law, that is, the state's authority must be legitimately used.

One important aspect of legitimacy has been the product of developments in the law regarding the rights of minorities, such as people with physical disabilities. It is now generally believed that legitimacy is undermined if the state shows a disregard for the political commitments that underwrite a free and democratic society. In particular, a disregard for the social commitment to equality, especially when manifested by arbitrary, irrational, or discriminatory policies prejudicing the interests of an identifiable group of people, undermines the legitimacy of the state's authority. Thus constitutional doctrine recognizes instances of the illegitimate and legally invalid use of authority, even where there is no doubt that the state possesses that authority.

This basic doctrine is reflected in the legal principles that could be called upon to assess the constitutionality of invasive AIDS measures. In the United States, any social response to the AIDS epidemic that infringed the guarantee of 'equal protection' would be subjected to strict judicial scrutiny.[16] The court would demand evidence that the 'proper purpose' of preserving public health was actually the goal of the proposed measures, rather than, say, quieting the unsupportable fears of the electorate, or pursuing a policy of harassing gays. The state would also be obliged to show that there is a rational connection between the objective of the measure and the means proposed to achieve it, and also that there are no other, less intrusive means available for achieving that end.

In Canada the governing law is the Charter of Rights and Freedoms, section 15 of which guarantees equality before the law and prohibits discrimination on various grounds, including mental and physical handicap. This provision firmly entrenches in the Canadian legal system the political value that all persons should be subject equally to whatever demands and burdens are imposed by law. Public health measures having the effect of disproportionately or unfairly burdening people with AIDS would thus be constitutionally suspect.

Were a particular AIDS measure to be challenged, a Canadian court would likely also investigate its professed purpose, and whether it was the least restrictive means available. Having done so, and having found that the measure violated the guarantee of equal treatment, the court would then be directed to section 1 of the Charter. Here it would consider whether this infringement of equality counts as a limitation that, in the language of the section, is 'reasonable and can be demonstrably justified in a free and democratic society'. Our courts have strongly suggested that considerations of cost, administrative expediency, or quieting public fears do not alone constitute demonstrable justifications; rather, the ultimate purpose behind the equality-infringing measure must itself be consistent with the values that allow all individuals to live their lives as free and equal citizens.[17] As before, the thrust of this requirement is that, at a minimum, sound medical evidence must be presented in support of the necessity of the public-health measure at issue.

From a legal point of view, then, if AIDS is understood as a handicapping condition, the social response to the AIDS epidemic must embody a rational respect for medical and other scientific evidence, possess a clearly enunciated purpose, be open to public scrutiny and debate, and show a commitment to avoiding unnecessary restrictions on the rights and interests of those with the disease. In effect, these are the law's guidelines for assessing the legitimacy of the use of the state's authority to deal with the AIDS epidemic.

And, as is not infrequently the case, guidelines imposed by the law reflect good sense, clarified and made practically feasible. For their purpose is not to outlaw all public-health measures, honestly and reasonably believed to be necessary in order to meet a health emergency, that happen to infringe or limit the rights of handicapped individuals. Rather, these guidelines ensure that attempts to respond to genuine and serious public health threats are medically necessary and do not needlessly violate the core political values that underwrite a free and democratic community.

Consider how these legal guidelines might help to clarify and resolve the basic tension between the effectiveness of health measures and the sacrifices they demand. Because of our political commitment to equality, the ultimate goal of our social response to AIDS must be to protect the legitimate interests of *everyone*. Thus people who have AIDS are protected from unwarranted infringements of equal protection, as well as from ill-conceived measures motivated by misinformation or fear. At the same time, as individuals with a contagious disease, people with AIDS do not have a legitimate interest in preventing any measure that is medically necessary to prevent the spread of the disease. As a rule, in other words, duties as well as rights are tied to disabilities.

The interests of those who are not HIV-infected are also best protected by a rational, and medically sound, response to the disease. In addition, it is in their interest to ensure that the rights of people with AIDS are protected, since, given the nature of the disease, there is no guarantee that they will not become members of that handicapped minority. Finally, it is not a legitimate interest of this majority that the social response to the AIDS epidemic be irrational, duplicitous, or discriminatory, or otherwise undermine unnecessarily the core political values of equality and liberty.

It is now easy to see why the objection mentioned earlier is fundamentally mistaken. A social response to AIDS that sets its standard of medical rationality at the level of medical certainty undermines the social commitment to equality, as it utterly pre-empts consideration of the interests of a specific minority. Given that such a social response would embody the claim that as a society we are unwilling to allow *any* level of risk for the sake of accommodating our political values, it would be illegitimate for the state to exercise its authority in this manner. And finally, such a policy would be both irrational and imprudent; it would cater to biases and fuel paranoia, greatly increase the likelihood of stigmatization, and make every unfounded fear a potential basis for a health measure.

CONCLUSION

Emphasizing the dimension of AIDS as a disability and handicap is helpful not merely because it avoids the distortions raised when issues of sexual morality dominate, but also because it enables us to tap the resources of the growing body of law involving disability. Of course, the legal principles and tests that govern this law have evolved in response to specific, interpersonal conflicts of interest and we must be cautious when we use them as guidelines for policy formation. And, of course, these principles and tests leave many practical questions unanswered: What level of risk is 'sufficient'? When are accommodations unreasonable? What state goals and purposes are proper? How do we determine the least restrictive alternative means? Still, it is often the case for policy issues of the complexity of those raised by AIDS that any assistance in knowing where to begin, what questions to ask, and what is really at stake is a great assistance indeed.

NOTES

[1]This perception is mirrored in many academic treatments of AIDS. The recent collection *AIDS: Ethics and Public Policy*, edited by Christine Pierce and Donald VanDeVeer (Belmont, CA: Wadsworth, 1988), for example, is almost entirely devoted to a discussion of sexual autonomy and related issues.

[2]The development of a metaphoric image of a disease, and so the creation of the social context of an epidemic, have been explored in Susan Sontag's powerful and justly influential treatment of disease in *Illness and Metaphor* (New York: Vintage Books, 1979); see as well her recent companion volume, *AIDS and Its Metaphors* (New York: Farrar, Straus, Giroux, 1988).

[3]See *International Classification of Impairments, Disabilities, and Handicaps: A Manual of Classification Relating to the Consequences of Diseases* (Geneva: World Health Organization, 1980), p. 28. The World Health Organization also defines an 'impairment' as 'any loss or abnormality of psychological, physiological, or anatomical structure or function' (p. 27). Although there are important differences between a disability and an impairment, inasmuch as AIDS is both no harm is done by conflating the two notions here.

[4]See the 'Denver Principles', the statement of the aims of the People With AIDS empowerment movement, set out in William B. Rubenstein, 'Law and Empowerment: The Idea of Order in the Time of AIDS', *Yale Law Journal* 98 (1989): 975, 990-4.

[5]The legal significance of this point was first developed by A. Leonard, 'Employment Discrimination Against Persons with AIDS', *University of Dayton Law Review* 10 (1985): 681.

[6]In the United States Supreme Court case of *School Board of Nassau County, Florida v. Arline* 480 US 273 (1987), a case involving a woman with tuberculosis who was fired from her job because she might be contagious, Mr Justice Brennen, writing for

the majority, said: 'Arline's contagiousness and her physical impairment each resulted from the same underlying condition, tuberculosis. It would be unfair to allow an employer to seize upon the distinction between the effects of a disease on others and the effects of a disease on a patient and use that distinction to justify discriminatory treatment.'

[7] I am presupposing what has come to be called the 'holistic' analysis of health and disease, the merits of which have been persuasively set out by Lennart Nordenfelt in *On the Nature of Health* (Dordrecht, Netherlands: Reidel Publishing Co., 1987).

[8] For a similar argument see Philip N. Bryden and Brian N. Jarrett 'AIDS, Employment Discrimination and the B.C. Human Rights Act', *Canadian Human Rights Reporter* 9 (1988), C/88-7.

[9] *Acquired Immunodeficiency Syndrome (AIDS): Policy Adopted by the Canadian Human Rights Commission* (May 1988) and *Ontario Human Rights Commission Policy on AIDS* (November 1985). See as well *Biggs v. Hudson, Canadian Human Rights Reporter* 9 (1988), D/5391, D/5395: 'Based upon the foregoing law and authorities, I find that any person who belongs to groups widely regarded as especially vulnerable to HIV infection but who are not HIV infected or whose HIV status is unknown ("high risk" groups) may be protected under the term "physical disability" in the [Human Rights] Act. Similarly, any person who associates with persons in the groups described above or those who are seropositive may be protected under the term "physical disability" in the Act.'

[10] Another situation that has arisen (more often in the United States than Canada) involves HIV-infected children who have been removed from school because of fears of contagion. In the United States, the Education for All Handicapped Children Act, 20 U.S.C. (1986) provides parents and educators with fairly clear guidelines for dealing with these troubling cases. In Canada, no such legislation exists and the situation is legally unclear.

[11] My scenario roughly follows the case of Eric Smith, a Shelburne County, Nova Scotia, teacher who was removed from the classroom and reassigned to non-teaching duties when a medical secretary disclosed that he had tested positive for the AIDS virus; the case was never litigated. (Cf. the United States case of *Chalk v. U.S. District Court Central California* 840 F. 2d 701 (9th Cir. 1988).) I am following here the analysis provided by Derek J. Jones and N. Colleen Sheppard in 'AIDS and Disability Employment Discrimination in and Beyond the Classroom', *Dalhousie Law Journal* 12 (1989): 103.

[12] Such is the wording of the exception found in the Ontario Human Rights Code, S.O. 1981, c. 53, as am., section 16(1).

[13] See Royal Society of Canada, *AIDS: A Perspective for Canadians (Summary Report and Recommendations)* (1988); David Spurgeon, *Understanding AIDS: A Canadian Strategy* (Toronto: Key Porter, 1988), and Canadian Medical Association, 'A CMA Position: Acquired Immunodeficiency Syndrome', *Canadian Medical Association Journal* 140 (1989): 64A.

[14] See the US Public Health Service, Centers for Disease Control, 'Guidelines for Prevention of Transmission of Human Immunodeficiency Virus and Hepatitis B

Virus to Health Care and Public Safety Workers' (Feb. 1989), and Canadian Federal Centre for AIDS, 'Occupational Exposure to the Human Immunodeficiency Virus Among Health Care Workers in Canada', *Canadian Medical Association Journal* 140 (1 March 1989): 503.

[15]In Canada, the general federal Parliament power of 'peace, order, and good government', coupled with its criminal law jurisdiction under section 91(27) of the British North America Act, 1868, authorizes it to pass legislation regarding health, including emergency legislation to deal with an epidemic.

[16]See the discussion of US equal-protection law in Note, 'The Constitutional Rights of AIDS Carriers', *Harvard Law Review* 99 (1987): 1274.

[17]I am following here the analysis of section 1 by Lorraine Eisenstat Weinrib in 'The Supreme Court of Canada and Section One of the Charter', *The Supreme Court Law Review* 10 (1988): 469.

AIDS AND WOMEN:
THE (HETERO)SEXUAL POLITICS
OF HIV INFECTION

———

CHRISTINE OVERALL

As of 7 May 1990, 211 women and 26 female children in Canada had developed Acquired Immunodeficiency Syndrome. Of these, 154 had died.[1] These figures may well under-represent the numbers of female Canadians with 'full-blown' AIDS, since the full spectrum of AIDS-related diseases in women often goes unrecognized as such.[2] Yet in North America, despite – or perhaps because of – an admirable concern to avoid the endemic homophobia typically aroused by stories about AIDS, most commentators continue to regard it as pre-eminently an infection of men,[3] and subscribe to the view that women are of interest not so much for their own sake but by virtue of their connection with men and children who are or may be infected.[4] Women are depicted 'not as individuals but merely as vectors of virus transmission'.[5]

Hence, while progressive commentators have been most concerned to combat gay-negative elements in AIDS policies and treatments, little attention has been paid to misogynous themes in AIDS policies, commentary, and education, which are rendered virtually invisible by the almost-exclusive focus on men.[6] Despite the growing incidence of AIDS and HIV-positivity in

27

women,[7] the situation of men with AIDS is usually taken to be the norm, and the issues that concern women – particularly with respect to reproduction and sexuality – are regarded as specialized, marginal, and less significant.[8] Implicit in the fact that less attention is paid to the manifestations and effects of AIDS in women[9] is the assumption that women's illnesses – and indeed, women themselves – are less important than men. In a patriarchal culture these values and assumptions are hardly surprising, but making them explicit may go some way towards rendering AIDS policies and practices less sexist.

Focusing primarily upon North American culture, this paper examines some ways in which social responses to, treatments of, and education about AIDS and about persons who have AIDS or who are HIV–positive reflect attitudes and practices that are oppressive to women. Discussion will be chiefly confined to issues pertaining to the sexual transmission of AIDS, since this means of infection is responsible for at least 59 per cent of AIDS cases in Canadian women.[10] Three themes will be explored: AIDS and gender stereo-types; AIDS and social inequality; and AIDS and sexual essentialism. My concern is not only with the examination of AIDS representations,[11] but with the exposure and assessment of the values that structure current thinking and feeling about AIDS. Thus the focus is not so much on women themselves (a group far too diverse to support casual generalizations), but on some of the norms that shape beliefs about and attitudes towards women.

AIDS AND GENDER STEREOTYPES

The social construction of the AIDS crisis provides a dramatization and reinforcement of some stereotypical gender constructs about women, partic-ularly with respect to women's procreative and sexual activities. Ironically, despite its singular dangers and debilitating effects, reactions to AIDS func-tion to confirm cultural givens about the allegedly eternal nature of Woman. These stereotypes – woman as nurturer and mother, or as seductress and prostitute – virtually always have two characteristics: they are constructed in terms of the extremes of good and bad, natural and unnatural;[12] and they serve to limit women's autonomy.

As mothers or potential mothers, women who are HIV–positive are believed to be of concern not so much for their own sake as for the sake of their fetuses or children.[13] Their significance is not for themselves, as persons whose lives have been drastically disrupted by a potentially fatal infection, but rather for their procreative and nurturing capacities, and the dark under-side of that nurturance, the ability to affect fetuses in utero and infants via breast milk.[14] 'Public recognition that women are susceptible to HIV disease – that women die from AIDS – has come almost by accident, secondhand to the rising number of babies with AIDS.'[15] As a result, in the United States women of childbearing age have been typically excluded from trials of new drug therapies for persons who are HIV-infected,[16] even though the drugs may subsequently be marketed for both men and women. Moreover, policy recommendations sometimes stress measures – such as mandatory prenatal testing without informed consent,[17] coercive abortion counselling, automatic Caesarean sections in the largely unsubstantiated hope of reducing the likelihood of fetal infection,[18] and loss of child custody – that deny women's reproductive autonomy and focus solely either upon the protection of fetal and infant well-being, or upon the elimination of another potential person with AIDS.[19] Katherine Franke has raised concerns about whether HIV-transmission may come to be considered a new form of so-called 'prenatal abuse', or whether failure to take still-experimental drugs for HIV-positivity during pregnancy may come to be grounds for accusations of 'prenatal neglect'.[20] Another possible spectre is the promotion of sterilization as the 'answer' to the problems of HIV-positive women of reproductive age.[21] This is not unthinkable, given the view of at least one author that HIV-positive women who do not abort are 'selfish' people who 'don't want to be alone in dying'.[22] And in an otherwise sympathetic paper, Nora Kizer Bell states that

> a prospective mother might be said to have an obligation to any potential child to spare it a certain and gruesome death, a prospective mother might be said to have an obligation to ensure and protect her own health for as long as she can (both for her own sake as well as for the sake of others, including the unborn fetus), and a prospective mother might be said to have an obligation to society not to bear children for whom society may have to provide.[23]

Bell concludes: 'While I do not believe that mandatory testing is either morally appropriate or enforceable, I do believe that it is morally irresponsible to argue in this case for preserving women's rights to reproductive choice', especially since, according to Bell, the fetus has not consented to exposing itself to the risk of HIV infection.[24] She regards the HIV-positive woman who fails to abort as more morally culpable than an infected person who knowingly donates blood. Thus HIV infection is being cited as a new justification for exerting control over women's fertility and reducing women's reproductive autonomy.

Ironically, some of the same people who advocate non-consensual prenatal testing are also willing to contemplate the possibility of women's risking HIV infection in order to become pregnant by their partners:

> One special case may be mentioned here: that of the seronegative woman whose sexual partner is seropositive. In this case, a woman may have to consider incurring the risk of becoming HIV positive herself to become pregnant; but she may judge this risk to be worthwhile to preserve something substantial from a relationship of love cut short by illness.[25]

It is extraordinary that these writers are willing to accept for women the risk of life-threatening illness in order to achieve pregnancy – and in particular, pregnancy with a specific man – rather than to recommend that such women make use of donor insemination using sperm that has been screened for HIV-positivity. This demonstrates that unexamined pronatalism – a mainstay of 'women's place' in the past – may also play a role in the spread of HIV infection to women.[26]

The Woman-as-Mother stereotype is further accentuated in recent media depictions of women as primarily nurturers of those who are HIV-positive.[27] Women are featured as the devoted mothers of infected adult sons and the faithful wives of infected husbands – and sometimes as lesbian comrades-in-arms of gay men with HIV.[28] Not surprisingly, there is no comparable cultural image of men as caregivers to women who are HIV-positive. Sometimes, also, women are portrayed as failing to fulfil their roles as nurturers, as for example when they are depicted as abandoning their HIV-infected infants.[29] And sometimes, also, women's nurturing role is treated not with respect but with an attitude close to resentment and contempt:

> One of the sadder moral side effects of the AIDS crisis is the number of men, stricken in their prime and deprived of medical insurance by forced unem-ployment, who have had to return to their *frequently bewildered mothers and alien environments* to be nursed through the final months of their suffering. Effec-tively denied the possibility of creating his own nurturing family, the son experiences the *final humiliation* of being treated again as a child. . . .[30]

No understanding is expressed here for the possible chagrin of the woman who finds herself 'having' to return to the long-finished role of mother, and who experiences the 'humiliation' of having that work resented by its very recipient.[31]

At the same time, the social construction of HIV infection may have pow-erful effects on women's self-image as mothers, for it threatens the standard view of women as reproducers. 'Abstaining from sex, which amounts to abstaining from having babies, is an unlikely solution for a woman who may find in children her sole source of love and self-worth, perhaps her sole hold on a man upon whom she depends for money.'[32] As a result, such women may rely on a kind of lottery mentality which says that while their chances of having an infected infant are high, there is also some chance that the baby will be healthy: to a woman with few other benefits in her life, this risk may well seem worth taking.

As many commentators have pointed out, HIV transmission is often inter-preted in terms of innocence and blame.[33] Sexually active people are held responsible for acquiring sexually transmitted diseases: a woman must there-fore be regarded as either the innocent recipient or the guilty transmitter of infection.[34] Assigning guilt and affixing blame serve to increase the isolation of women with HIV infection, who in any case often lack the kinds of support usually available to persons living with AIDS (PLWAs) who are members of gay communities.[35] As sexual beings, women are seen either as passive and good victims of HIV transmission from men (pure virgins affected through artificial insemination by infected sperm, and faithful wives/partners contaminated by sexually deviant husbands) or as actively evil transmitters (prostitutes or stereotypically 'loose' women) of disease to men. In today's cultural climate, the presence of AIDS is ineluctably associated with sexual activity; in patriarchal either/or terms, women must be perceived either as sexual victims who have acquired the infection from rapacious men, or as sexual temptresses who transmit infection to innocent men who are overcome by their blandishments.

Many writers have pointed out that real social concern about HIV infection did not materialize until its potential 'spread to heterosexuals' was recognized.[36] What is less often pointed out is that concern for the 'spread to heterosexuals' has mostly been manifest in concern for the spread to heterosexual *men*, not heterosexual women. The expressed fear is that HIV will spread from women to men, allegedly through prostitution.[37] Interestingly, there is evidence that some HIV-positive men may be inclined to claim that their infection came from a female prostitute, in order to cover up its real origins: sex with a man, or IV drug use.[38] Definitions of manhood are not only consistent with but enhanced by buying sex from a woman, but they are compromised by consensual sex with another male.

Thus, after a long history in which prostitutes have been held responsible for spreading sexually transmitted diseases, AIDS has been taken to provide a new and more powerful reason to prosecute and punish sex workers, while protecting their customers not only from legal repercussions, but even from public recognition of their resort to paid sex.[39] 'The "public" appears not to be concerned about whether prostitutes themselves die, but whether they transmit the virus to their male customers, who then pass it on to "innocent" women and children.'[40] Clear evidence of this set of priorities can be found in Ruth Macklin's statement: 'Public health concerns focus on two groups of potential *victims* [of prostitutes]: men who patronize prostitutes (including male prostitutes); and infants born of seropositive female prostitutes.'[41] This reaction overlooks the very low rates of infection among North American prostitutes,[42] the lack of evidence of infection of customers by prostitutes,[43] and sex workers' own motivation to protect themselves.[44]

The negative moral notion of promiscuity is applied differently to women than to heterosexual men: while such men are said to be 'sexually active', women are are said to be 'promiscuous'. As Pierce and VanDeVeer point out, the term 'promiscuous' is often used to mean not merely 'having a large number of sexual partners' but also 'having *too many* sexual partners'.[45] Unfortunately, the association of condom use with 'promiscuity' and prostitution, with infection and the prevention of infection, may be precisely what precludes its use by many women. 'Some women . . . worry that if you're requesting safe sex, you're essentially saying (a) that you're a slut who might be *spreading* disease; (b) that you suspect him of being homosexual and/or an addict; or (c) that you resent his sleeping with other women.'[46] Yet it is not necessarily the number of partners that increases the risk of HIV infection, but rather the kinds of sexual activities engaged in: a woman could easily be infected by one HIV-positive individual with whom she has a long-term unprotected monogamous relationship.[47] This fact is obscured when estimates of prevalence of HIV infection in a defined group are confused with explications of the causes of infection.

AIDS AND SOCIAL INEQUALITY

At the same time that social understandings of AIDS and HIV infection are reinforcing painfully familiar gender stereotypes, some approaches to AIDS education and prevention are paradoxically assuming a non-existent 'level playing field' for women and men that obscures both the public and private inequities in power that continue to define women and men and their relationships. For example, discussions of AIDS education typically do not recognize that heterosexuality is a social institution, not merely a private and individual sexual preference, that rape is a pervasive male practice, and that much heterosexual activity is coercive. The emphasis on safer sex, including the use of condoms, on co-operative practices such as voluntarily informing sex partners when one is infected, and on confidentiality and protection of privacy in treatment of AIDS patients, may overestimate the extent of male/female equality, the extent of women's free choice with respect to their heterosexual activities, and the degree to which men are willing to inform and protect their female partners by using condoms and permitting and facilitating voluntary notification of sexual partners.[48]

Thus Ronald Bayer, Carol Levine, and Susan M. Wolf correctly remark that 'there is a moral obligation for antibody-positive individuals to notify their sexual partners, especially when their partners have no reason to suspect that they have had contact with an individual at risk for HIV infection',[49] but they fail to acknowledge the sexual politics that makes heterosexual women and men unequal moral partners in sexual relationships. As Ruth Macklin wisely comments:

> Most people lie, at least sometimes, about trivial as well as important matters. If women were to ask prospective or even regular sex partners whether they are HIV-positive, it is folly to think that those partners would always reply truthfully even if they knew the answer. If they have not altered their own sexual behavior, or if they have not voluntarily disclosed their status to a woman before she asks, it is naïve to think that they would answer a direct question truthfully.

However, Macklin then draws a surprising conclusion: 'Women could, then, adopt the safer policy of insisting that all sex partners use condoms.'[50] The likelihood of male mendacity with respect to sex and AIDS is being amply documented.[51] It is equally 'naïve' to suppose that those men who may lie, who do not know their HIV status, and who have not yet changed their sexual behaviour, will readily comply with a woman's 'insistence' on their using condoms. Moreover, rapists presumably do not inform their victims of their HIV status,[52] and women and children are not able to ask the men who sexually assault them to use a condom.

Some AIDS groups have been concerned about cases in which HIV-positive men have been charged with assault for having unprotected sex without informing their partners of their medical condition.[53] The argument is that sexually active people should not assume their partners are not infected; responsibility for sexual safety rests on both partners, and women, once again, should insist their partners use condoms.[54] Indeed, Richard Mohr suggests, confidently, 'Each person on *his* own – without state coercion – can get the protection from the disease that *he* wants through *his* own actions'.[55] However, as Lisa McCaskell has pointed out:

> Many men don't want to talk openly with women about sexual behaviour and history. They may not want to tell about previous homosexual experiences or injection drug use. They may not want to divulge information about previous lovers. Many women do not feel free to ask their male lovers about these things and often they may not want to know the answers. Talking about sex may be particularly difficult for some women for whom cultural patterns of subservience to husbands is basic to the relationship. This may also be true for older women who have been married for years and who have never openly questioned their partners' fidelity or admitted their own affairs.[56]

Thus the problem with Mohr's statement is that norms for mostly egalitarian gay relationships cannot necessarily be applied to mostly non-egalitarian heterosexual relationships. As Larry Gostin and William J. Curran note, 'sexual acts are *not* wholly consensual if the infected person fails to inform his partner of the substantial risk to health'.[57] Women who do not know their partner's HIV status, who indeed may not even know that their partner engages in risk-related activities, do not give unconstrained consent to heterosexual activity; and their capacity to obtain the information that would enable them to make an informed choice about their sexual partners and activities is itself constrained by the conditions of limited power and freedom under which they operate.

Women are not supposed, and often not allowed, to take the lead in sex, or to set the conditions governing their sexual interactions;[58] in fact, as accumulating evidence grimly confirms, because of women's internalized oppression, they often cannot even say no to a sexual 'invitation'. Just as, in the recent past, merely telling women that they must take responsibility for birth control in no way empowered them to attain reproductive control over their lives, so also telling women that they must take responsibility for sexual safety, through condom use or non-penetrative sex, in no way empowers them to assume sexual control. Simply assigning the responsibility to women fails to challenge the power inequities between women and men, and may even exacerbate them, in cases where men react violently to this curtailment of their sexual liberty.[59] And many women are not in a position simply to leave men who cannot be 'persuaded' to practise safer sex.[60]

Indeed, for women, the notion of 'safer sex' may be little more than a contradiction in terms. Contraceptive safety and efficacy have been notoriously difficult to achieve, even – or especially – in this era of high-tech contraception. Women might be forgiven for being suspicious about the much-touted claim that, with a life-threatening viral infection in the offing, safer sex is now an achievable goal,[61] especially since, in heterosexual activities, women may be more at risk for HIV infection than men because sperm is one of the main transmitters of HIV. As Bell notes, there is also a regrettable absence of 'research efforts to develop better barriers to transmission for women'.[62] But even if such barriers were developed, there would still be the matter of eliciting the co-operation – or at least acquiescence – of male partners in their use. In fact, women may be encouraged to see 'risky business' as an inevitable part of what is titillating about sexual encounters.

Recent bioethical discussions of the issue of confidentiality also appear to assume an implausible male/female parity, with a prime emphasis on the preservation of personal sexual privacy and the recommendation of individual responsibility as the predominant moral themes.[63] The problem is that promoting these values is seldom adequate to compensate for the social effects of sexism, and indeed, promotion of privacy as a pre-eminent value has often served to protect men's sexual access to and violation of women and children rather than women and children themselves. Nora Kizer Bell argues that efforts to 'develop policy that would be responsible to the privacy rights of persons with AIDS' have 'had the effect of slowing public health efforts to institute partner notification'.[64] An article by Morton Winston and Sheldon H. Landesman raises concerns about the protection of the confidentiality of a bisexual HIV-positive husband, at the expense of his female partner's need to know.[65] While pointing out, with some justification, that violations of confidentiality would cause a decline in the numbers of persons seeking testing and counselling, both commentators entirely ignore the sexual politics of marriage and heterosexual relationships. One commentator is chiefly worried about the possibility that the physician of such a man might be sued by one partner or the other; the other complacently remarks that infection of the woman 'may be the cost that society pays if it wishes to implement public health measures to minimize the spread of the virus'.[66] While confidentiality remains an essential ethical principle in medical practice, it is also important to notice both who is protected by confidentiality and who pays the price for it. In this sort of case, it is not some faceless and amorphous 'society' that suffers; it is real women.

Likewise, Richard Mohr rather contemptuously dismisses ethical concerns about the effect on women of respect for confidentiality, stating that

> the person who gets AIDS through sexual contact . . . actively participates in the very action that harms him [*sic*] and his deeds are properly said to be a contributory cause of the harms that come to him. He is not a victim. . . . Only the most compelling state interest could justify overriding the right to privacy exampled in the patient–doctor relation. Yet saving people *from themselves* is necessarily a weaker state interest than saving people *from each other*. The privacy right in the AIDS case is therefore not properly overridden by a state interest in protecting a wife from herself. . . . That popular support for the doctor telling the wife is so overwhelming . . . suggests that America still does not view wives as people.[67]

It is of course naïve to regard women, even those who are wives, as mere helpless and vulnerable victims. But neither are they yet able to be the social equals of men. To recognize the ways in which women can be deceived, exploited, and harmed by those to whom they are wed is not to fail to see wives as people (though many in 'America' may indeed fail to do that); it is to recognize that the heterosexual institution of marriage may not work to the advantage of women in the way that it can work to the advantage of men.

In view of the concern expressed by bioethicists about preservation of the confidentiality of HIV-positive men, it is surprising to find suggestions by some commentators about notifying the male partners of HIV-positive women. Almond and Ulanowsky claim, 'As far as physicians are concerned, the situation could be regarded as one in which a breach of confidentiality would be *justified* where a woman was unwilling to take any kind of action herself. . . .'[68] Indeed, in a recent case in the Northwest Territories, the Medical Officer of Health threatened to reveal the identity of a woman who had tested positive for HIV.[69] Yet the outcome for a woman whose male partners are informed of her HIV-positive status against her will is potentially more perilous than the outcome for a bisexual man whose partners are informed of his HIV-positive status. For she runs the risk of abandonment, economic impoverishment, and possibly even physical assault.[70]

Christine Pierce and Donald VanDeVeer dryly remark, without further comment, 'There has been no criticism by feminists to the effect that because AIDS is primarily a disease of males [at least in North America] . . . men, by and large, are responsible for spreading it.'[71] This is, of course, a dangerously misleading statement. In statistical terms, more men than women transmit HIV in North America – and they transmit it to women as well as to other men. This is not to say that men do so deliberately, or even, in many cases, knowingly. Paula Treichler pours scorn, with good reason, on AIDS discourse by and about women that embraces the 'us' and 'them' division, 'advising "us" (women) to protect ourselves from "them" (men).'[72] Nevertheless, recognizing and resisting the scapegoating of gay and bisexual men and indeed any man who is HIV-positive must not be incompatible with a concern for the interests of women who may be affected by their various connections and relationships with HIV-positive men. It should also be accompanied by a recognition of the ways in which socially sanctioned male access to women's bodies makes women particularly vulnerable to HIV infection, through their economic dependence on men, through enculturated submissiveness to men, and through male assault and sexual abuse.

AIDS AND SEXUAL ESSENTIALISM

The foregoing themes indicate an asymmetry, in contemporary North American responses to AIDS, with respect to women and men: gender differences are emphasized and exaggerated; but power differences are denied or overlooked. Both the gender stereotyping of women and the masking of power inequities between women and men are founded upon an essentialist conception of women's and men's natures, and especially of the character of human sexuality and sexual interactions, exacerbated by the categorization of kinds of sexual persons supposedly at greater or lesser risk for contracting HIV.

Sexual definitions are limited by essentialist concepts of gender and sexual orientation – concepts that purport to reflect the true, inherent nature of individuals of a particular sex and sexual orientation. Both the media, which reify groups of allegedly high-risk persons[73] such as gay males, and gay-rights advocates themselves seem committed to defining persons in terms of who they are rather than what they do.[74] But this approach obfuscates questions of probability with questions of causation. Thus women who sleep with men who regard themselves as heterosexual but who have had sexual relationships with other men may falsely believe that their partners cannot be infectious. Or, a woman who now defines herself as lesbian may overlook her own previous sexual activities with men, and, once again, falsely regard herself as not vulnerable to HIV infection. Without in any way denigrating the value of identity politics in gay/lesbian liberation struggles, it must also be recognized that this commitment to identity sometimes tends to obscure rather than illuminate the kinds of risks that women may in fact face.

The problem is not merely, as many commentators have tirelessly pointed out, that 'gay' is equated with 'AIDS', so that those who are heterosexual and those who are lesbian have mistakenly seen themselves as not at risk. The problem is also that the categories themselves are seen as impermeable identity-boxes, a view that obscures the real variety of people's sexual activities, sexual partners, and sexual self-identifications.[75] In addition, at least in common parlance, those identity-boxes themselves are limited in number, by what Jan Zita Grover refers to as 'the balkanization of sexual desire'.[76] While AIDS epidemiologists often recognize that some men are bisexual, there is not a common and accepted cultural use of the concept of bisexual man, let alone bisexual woman. Thus 'sexual desire is parcelled into two exclusive realms, the homosexual and heterosexual "communities", with the bisexual – understood as a homosexual *posing* as a heterosexual – acting as the secret conveyor of the diseases of the former to the healthy bodies of the latter'.[77] The fact that homophobia reinforced by AIDS-related panic also ends up hurting lesbians is seldom recognized except by lesbians themselves.[78]

Moral systems that stress unfettered sexual freedom, the quantity rather than the quality of sexual experience, and the primacy of (male) desire continue to influence contemporary thinking about AIDS.[79] While women are clearly unfairly stereotyped by allegations of 'promiscuity', it does not follow that they are well-served by defences of heterosexual non-monogamy and sexual 'freedom', since these so often support male privilege rather than female freedom. When Douglas Crimp argues that 'gay male promiscuity should be seen . . . as a positive model of how sexual pleasures might be pursued by and granted to everyone if those pleasures were not confined within the narrow limits of institutionalized sexuality',[80] it is hard to believe that these pleasures would be available to women, because that would entail so radical a reorganization of sexual roles and gender power. The defence of large numbers of sexual partners often turns out to mean large numbers of partners for men; this usually requires access to women's bodies, but does not necessarily support women's own sexual self-determination. In any case, the notion that sexual activity is the main or the only route to closeness and intimacy requires re-examination; it may be that the real human need for physical contact gets confused with limited forms of sexual gratification.

The sexual liberals' emphasis on sexual freedom is in ironic juxtaposition with a growing sexual conservatism that emphasizes abstinence and monogamy, and assumes that certain activities are inherently unnatural and wrong. The misleading emphasis, in public education about AIDS, on the significance of monogamy as preventive behaviour appears to confirm the old stereotype that every woman's destiny is lifelong coupling with one man. As Erika Parsa observes, 'This puts a lot of pressure on relationships. . . . The fidelity solution to the AIDS epidemic acts almost as a threat, coercing couples to stay together.'[81] Thus the only two possibilities currently offered to women seem to be dangerous sexual activity, mitigated only partially through condom use – if the latter can be achieved – or 1950s-style lifelong monogamy with a 'safe' partner. Are there other possibilities for women? Most AIDS education so far has given little indication. Significantly, it seldom recognizes low-risk sex with women as an alternative to more risky heterosexual activities.

In AIDS education and prevention programs, (hetero)sexual intercourse (penetration) is regarded as the primary or even the only form of sexual activity. Much state-mandated AIDS education 'presumes that the only type of sex that people can have is unprotected penile/vaginal intercourse, and that married people are somehow immune from infection'.[82] Real sexual behaviour, in this view, is limited to penetration, so that the apparently 'pro-sex' approach to some AIDS education primarily protects certain forms of sex, and assumes that penetrative sexual practices are impossible to change.[83] It therefore fails to promote women's sexual freedom and control:

> many brochures on 'safe sex' concentrate on describing ways to make the condom more palatable to the male sexual experience than they do either on ways to ensure the safety of the woman receptor or on sexual practices that are non-penetrative. The many public health messages recommending condom use have conveyed the impression that the male sexual experience is the primary focus.[84]

Male sexual desire is regarded as irrepressible and uncontrollable (the same assumption sometimes used to rationalize the occurrence of rape). For example, in an article on AIDS and state coercion, Richard Mohr argues that sexual activity is 'a natural object, not a product', and claims, ominously, that 'its frustration tends to sponsor aggression'.[85] Sexual access of men to women is regarded as the unquestionable foundation stone of 'human' sexual freedom and fulfilment. The exaggerated respect for male desire and the unquestioning acceptance of penetration feed cultural stereotypes of traditional masculinity.[86]

CONCLUSION

Contemporary forms of oppression and injustice make HIV infection not only a serious medical condition but also a life-threatening political problem for women. The case made here is not that current education, policies, and commentary about AIDS and HIV infection are all entirely mistaken, but rather that, insofar as they are derived from attention to the situations of men, they cannot be assumed to apply directly to women or to promote women's well-being. It is time to re-evaluate and reject those forms of AIDS education, policy-formation, and activism that simply support and reinforce oppressive gender stereotypes, limited sexual roles, and misogynist practices.

NOTES

I would like to thank the staff of the Kingston AIDS Project for their assistance.

[1] Federal Centre for AIDS, 'Surveillance Update: AIDS in Canada' (Ottawa 1990), p. 1.

[2] Diane Richardson, *Women and the AIDS Crisis*, new ed. (London: Pandora, 1989), p. 28.

[3] Julien S. Murphy, 'Women with AIDS: Sexual Ethics in an Epidemic', in Inge B.

Corless and Mary Pittman-Lindeman, eds, *AIDS: Principles, Practices, and Politics* (New York: Hemisphere, 1988), pp. 65-6.

[4]Paula A. Treichler, 'AIDS, Gender, and Biomedical Discourse: Current Contests for Meaning', in Elizabeth Fee and Daniel M. Fox, eds, *AIDS: The Burdens of History* (Berkeley: University of California Press, 1988), p. 215.

[5]Janet L. Mitchell, 'Women, AIDS, and Public Policy', *AIDS and Public Policy Journal* 3, 2 (1988): 50.

[6]Treichler, 'AIDS, Gender, and Biomedical Discourse', p. 193.

[7]Nora Kizer Bell, 'Women and AIDS: Too Little, Too Late?', *Hypatia* 4, 3 (Fall 1989): 3-6.

[8]One small but significant indicator of women's marginality in the AIDS epidemic is the fact that at the Queen's University Library, the keyword 'AIDS' calls up well over 1200 entries, whereas the phrase 'AIDS and Women' calls up exactly five.

[9]Chris Norwood, 'Alarming Rise in Deaths', *Ms.* 17, 1 (July 1988): 65, 67; Sue Halpern, 'AIDS: Rethinking the Risk', *Ms.* 17, 11 (May 1989): 80-1.

[10]Federal Centre for AIDS, p. 4.

[11]This approach is exemplified in Douglas Crimp, ed., *AIDS: Cultural Analysis/ Cultural Activism* (Cambridge, MA: MIT Press, 1988).

[12]For examples, see Paula A. Treichler, 'AIDS, Homophobia, and Biomedical Discourse: An Epidemic of Signification', in ibid., pp. 63-4.

[13]A good example is Esther Chachkes's 'Women and Children with AIDS', in Carl G. Leukefeld and Manuel Fimbres, eds, *Responding to AIDS: Psychosocial Initiatives* (Silver Spring, MD: National Association of Social Workers, 1987), pp. 51-64, which, despite its title, focuses almost entirely on issues affecting children.

[14]Diane Richardson suggests that the alleged dangers of HIV infection via breast milk could conceivably be used by manufacturers of artificial infant formula to promote sales of their product (p. 61).

[15]Halpern, p. 87.

[16]Ibid., p. 86.

[17]Brenda Almond and Carole Ulanowsky, 'HIV and Pregnancy', *Hastings Center Report* 20, 2 (March/April 1990): 17.

[18]Ibid., pp. 18-19.

[19]Katherine Franke, 'Turning Issues Upside Down', in Ines Rieder and Patricia Ruppelt, eds, *AIDS: The Women* (San Francisco: Cleis Press, 1988), pp. 227-8.

[20]Ibid., p. 229.

[21]Mitchell, p. 51.

[22]Gregory E. Pence, *Classical Cases in Medical Ethics* (New York: McGraw-Hill, 1990), pp. 342-3.

[23]Bell, pp. 15-16.

[24]Ibid., p. 17.

[25]Almond and Ulanowsky, p. 18.

[26]See Richardson, p. 64. She points out that so-called 'surrogate' mothers hired to gestate infants for pay may run the risk of HIV infection if the semen is not tested (p. 60). It is also ironic that donor insemination, a means sought by some women to achieve pregnancy independent of the risks of heterosexual intercourse, is a perilous undertaking if the semen is not tested. See also Cheri Pies, 'Insemination: Something More to Consider', in Rieder and Ruppelt, eds, *AIDS: The Women*, pp. 139-42.

[27]Richardson, p. 130.

[28]Deborah Stone, 'A Selfish Kind of Giving', in Rieder and Ruppelt, eds, *AIDS: The Women*, pp. 143-50.

[29]Franke, p. 226.

[30]Richard D. Mohr, *Gays/Justice: A Study of Ethics, Society, and Law* (New York: Columbia University Press, 1988), p. 238, emphasis added.

[31]Richardson, pp. 140-4.

[32]Mary T. Schmich, 'Spreading the Word on Safe Sex', *Toronto Star* (27 July 1989): K1. See also Bell, pp. 14-15.

[33]Judith Wilson Ross, 'Ethics and the Language of AIDS', in Christine Pierce and Donald VanDeVeer, eds, *AIDS: Ethics and Public Policy* (Belmont, CA: Wadsworth, 1988), pp. 41-2.

[34]Treichler, 'AIDS, Gender, and Biomedical Discourse', p. 191.

[35]Darien Taylor, 'Testing Positive', *Healthsharing* 11, 2 (Spring 1990): 10.

[36]For example, Randy Shilts, *And the Band Played On: Politics, People, and the AIDS Epidemic* (New York: St Martin's Press, 1987).

[37]Ibid., p. 510.

[38]Ibid., p. 511.

[39]Richardson, p. 44.

[40]Debi Brock, 'Prostitutes are Scapegoats in the AIDS Panic', *Resources for Feminist Research/Documentation sur la recherche féministe* 18, 2 (June 1989): 13.

[41]Ruth Macklin, 'Predicting Dangerousness and the Public Health Response to AIDS', *Hastings Center Report* 16, 6, Special Supplement (December 1986), p. 22, emphasis added.

[42]Richardson, p. 42.

[43]Shilts, p. 513.

[44]Borck, p. 14.

[45]Christine Pierce and Donald VanDeVeer, 'General Introduction', in *AIDS: Ethics and Public Policy*, pp. 14-15.

[46]Lindsy Van Gelder, 'AIDS', *Ms.* 15, 10 (April 1987): 71, her emphasis.

[47]Richardson, p. 40.

[48]Bell, p. 12.

[49]Ronald Bayer, Carol Levine, and Susan M. Wolf, 'HIV Antibody Screening: An Ethical Framework for Evaluating Proposed Programs', in Tom L. Beauchamp and LeRoy Walters, eds, *Contemporary Issues in Bioethics* (Belmont, CA: Wadsworth, 1989), pp. 638-9.

[50]Macklin, p. 20.

[51]'Women and AIDS Project' (New York, Spring 1989), p. 19.

[52]Richardson points out that injuries inflicted during a rape may make transmission of HIV more likely (p. 48).

[53]It seems unlikely that many women will come forward to complain that they have had a sexual relationship with a man who failed to inform them of his HIV-positive status. It is well known that women are very fearful of reporting rape and sexual assault; they seldom boast about their consensual sexual relationships; and they are even less likely to speak publicly of activities associated with stigma in the way that HIV infection is.

[54]'AIDS Carrier Charged for Allegedly Having Sex Without Telling Partners', *Kingston Whig-Standard* (10 April 1989): 3.

[55]Richard D. Mohr, 'AIDS, Gays and State Coercion', *Bioethics* 1, 1 (January 1987): 48, emphasis added.

[56]Lisa McCaskell, 'We Are Not Immune: Women and AIDS', *Healthsharing* 9, 4 (Fall 1988): 16.

[57]Larry Gostin and William J. Curran, 'The Limits of Compulsion in Controlling AIDS', *Hastings Center Report* 16, 6, Special Supplement (December 1986): 28.

[58]Richardson, p. 85.

[59]Bell, p. 11.

[60]Schmich, p. K1.

[61]Bell, p. 11.

[62]Ibid.

[63]See Ronald Bayer, *Private Acts, Social Consequences: AIDS and the Politics of Public Health* (New York: Free Press, 1989), pp. 20-71.

[64]Bell, pp. 8-9.

[65]Morton Winston and Sheldon H. Landesman, 'AIDS and a Duty to Protect', *Hastings Center Report* 17, 1 (February 1987): 22-3.

[66]Ibid., p. 23.

[67]Mohr, *Gays/Justice*, pp. 227-8, fn. 23, his emphasis.

[68]Almond and Ulanowsky, p. 20.

[69]'Confidentiality Compromised', *Rites* 6, 10 (April 1990): 1.

[70]Halpern, p. 85.

[71]Pierce and VanDeVeer, p. 8.

[72]Treichler, 'AIDS, Gender, and Biomedical Discourse', p. 197; cf. p. 226.

[73]For example, the publication *On Balance* complains about CBC television's coverage of AIDS news that 'in promoting the theme that AIDS is not a gay disease, CBC obscured the fact that homosexual and bisexual men are most at risk. . . . CBC downplayed the gay role by mentioning AIDS' transmission through homosexual and bisexual sex in less than one percent of its coverage on transmission, despite the fact that 85.3 percent of AIDS patients contracted the disease through bisexual or homosexual intercourse' (National Media Archive, 'AIDS: Epidemiology, Fear, Education and Human Rights', *On Balance* 2, 7 [July/August 1989]: 2, 7). In this case, one medium is complaining about the failure of another medium to scapegoat certain alleged risk groups.

[74]Mary Louise Adams, 'Cindy Patton on Safer Sex, Community and Porn', *Rites* 5, 10 (April 1989): 11.

[75]Pierce and VanDeVeer, p. 10.

[76]Jan Zita Grover, 'AIDS: Keywords', in *AIDS: Cultural Analysis/Cultural Activism*, p. 21.

[77]Ibid., p. 21, her emphasis.

[78]Vada Hart, 'Lesbians and A.I.D.S.', *Gossip: A Journal of Lesbian Feminist Ethics* 2 (1986): 92-3; Grover, p. 25; Richardson, p. 68.

[79]See, for example, Douglas Crimp, 'How to Have Promiscuity in an Epidemic', in *AIDS: Cultural Analysis/Cultural Activism*, pp. 237-71.

[80]Ibid., p. 253.

[81]Erika Parsa, 'Caution Rather Than Panic', in Rieder and Ruppelt, eds, *AIDS: The Women*, p. 192.

[82]Franke, p. 232.

[83]Adams, p. 10.

[84]Bell, p. 11.

[85]Mohr, 'AIDS, Gays and State Coercion', p. 45.

[86]Richardson, p. 87.

AIDS, ETHICS AND RELIGION

___

WILLIAM P. ZION

The present emergence of AIDS as a threat to society poses an urgent need for reflection on the relation of illness to notions of sin and evil. Interpretations of illness as the consequence of sin are deeply embedded in the religious dimensions of North American society. For many Christians it has not been enough to consider AIDS as a physical evil brought on by the human immunodeficiency virus: they have identified AIDS as a punishment inflicted upon sinners by God. This view has been expressed not only by fundamentalist preachers such as Jerry Falwell but by prominent Roman Catholic spokesmen, the most notable being Archbishop John Foley, a curial official in Rome who identified AIDS as a 'sanction'. When asked if the archbishop was correct in his judgement, Pope John Paul II replied that 'it is hard to know the mind of God.'[1] Few others, however, have shown such hesitation in knowing God's mind. In a publication of the Evangelical Fellowship of Canada, for instance, the editor-in-chief, Brian C. Stiller, called AIDS 'a message to the world that humankind cannot violate God's laws without repercussions'.[2]

These reactions of the religious communities and churches are indicative of how large segments of society are responding to the threat of AIDS: by 'blaming the victim'. However illogical it may be, the afflicted persons themselves are seen as the cause of the disease. Despite the evidence that persons with AIDS in Africa are predominantly heterosexual and often include infants, a disease that threatens us all is blamed on homosexual 'promiscuity'. There has emerged a multitude of voices crying out for the repression of homosexuals and a quarantine for those infected with HIV.[3] The American psychiatrist Stuart Nichols has written of what lies behind these attitudes:

> Insight into the society's sexual anxiety is important beyond the understand-
> ing of AIDS. Psychiatrists must also understand that the impossible attempt to
> protect ourselves from our own sexual natures has dire consequences. Since
> the defense against our own homoerotic feeling requires that homosexuals be
> regarded as different, they are likely to be seen as inferior or even less human
> in some essential way. In troubled times they become ready targets for
> scapegoating.[4]

The search for a culprit to blame and punish not only serves as a way of assuring ourselves that we are not at fault, but allows us to imagine that elimination of the culprit will leave us safe and secure once more. The deep historical roots of this tendency in human society have been explored by the French literary critic René Girard,[5] who has identified the sacrifice of 'trouble-makers' as the core of religious practice – a means of healing society by destroying those who would threaten it.

The condemnation of homosexual men as deserving a death for which they themselves are to blame is very much a part of this and other religious traditions that have fed on anti-Semitism, racism, and sexism. Now vast numbers of Christians see AIDS as just recompense for those who do not abstain from all sexual activity outside of heterosexual marriage. According to this logic, lung cancer would be the punishment for the sin of smoking, and cyrrhosis of the liver the punishment for the sin of drinking alcohol. Yet most Christians have not judged the victims of these diseases in the harsh and uncompromising way they have condemned people with AIDS.

While it is true that the Hebrew Bible condemns a man to death if he lies with another man as with a woman (Lev. 18: 22) the same Bible also demands that a father kill his son if he is disobedient (Deut. 21: 18-21) – an injunction that is ignored as a cultural anachronism by believers who generally choose what they want from biblical law and dismiss what they do not want. Christians have long since followed St Paul in giving up adherence to most Mosaic law, distinguishing between ceremonial laws and natural laws, which remain perennially valid. While Protestants have sought to ground natural law in biblical teaching, Catholics have largely adopted the Stoic propensity to found it in orders of nature.

Moreover, St Paul's own supposed references to homosexuality are highly questionable. The words translated as 'homosexual' (*arsenokoitos* and *malakos*) in the Revised Standard Version of his epistles (1 Cor. 6: 9 and 1 Tim. 1: 10) are so difficult to translate that scholars are divided over their meanings. Indeed, most question whether they have anything at all to do with homosexual activity. For example, the traditional exegesis of the first chapter of the Letter to the Romans assumes that in it Paul makes a blanket condemnation of homosexuality. In fact it is idolatry that he condemns, and he cites Greek homosexuality only as an illustration of the consequences of idolatry among the Gentiles, a practice that, like eating forbidden food, is unclean and shameful. Paul's central point – to show how all human beings have sinned and need the grace and forgiveness of God – is completely negated when his portrayal of the consequences of idolatry is turned into a new version of the law. Ammunition for homophobia has been mined from these sources for two thousand years, despite the good news in the letters of Paul that all may be saved no matter what the depths of their sinfulness may be.

In fact, the homophobic interpretation of the AIDS epidemic is not only lacking in scriptural justification; it is also fundamentally inconsistent with the primacy of charity in biblical ethics. It is my wish in this paper to present an alternative interpretation based on principles that are equally deeply rooted in the Judaeo-Christian tradition.

First, however, it is important to consider why such interpretation is necessary at all. Susan Sontag, for example, has declared it imperative that illness be entirely freed from the bondage of metaphors – religious or secular – that lead to blaming the sick for their illness.[6] The problem with Sontag's approach is that it denies the possibility of learning anything from AIDS, apart from the advisability of practising 'safer sex'. The epidemic becomes merely an accident of biological history, to be corrected by prophylactic measures; then, presumably, the sexual behaviour that characterized urban life in capitalist societies can pick up where it left off.[7]

I suggest that stripping away the metaphors is not enough. Human beings need to find meaning – above all, when they are facing a potential death sentence – and AIDS is already being popularly interpreted in ways that can be countered only by alternative readings.

In contrast to these moralistic, paternalistic, punitive interpretations of AIDS, I suggest an interpretation built on non-violence, on compassion for the suffering and the dying, on the recognition of homosexuals as persons whom God has created, and on the acceptance of homosexual acts as moral as long as they are expressive of love between two persons and carried out without inflicting harm. The religious foundations of these attitudes are at least as deep as those of the punitive and homophobic. The link between the suffering and Christ himself is deeply embedded in the teachings of Jesus (Matt. 25: 36). The association between illness and sin is not a dominant one within the Jewish or Christian traditions. Jewish religious principles demand that we not judge anyone and always put ourselves in the place of the one that we are tempted to accuse,[8] and Jesus' basic maxim was 'judge not'. Homophobia is inherently violent, whereas the way of Christ is the rejection of all violence. How far we have come from the stance taken by Jesus is found in John 8: 1-11, the story of Jesus' intervention when a woman was about to be stoned to death for adultery: 'Let him who is without sin throw the first stone.'

If we are to use theological and moral metaphor creatively, we must overcome the inherently homophobic undertones in the natural law morality that condemns homosexual acts as of themselves immoral and evil. What is offered in this form of morality is a link between a theological teleology (whereby a moral norm is imposed by God's creation of the sexual faculties for purposes of procreation) and apodictic moral norms. Whatever does not orient itself to procreation is condemned as gravely evil. Since the context of procreation must be heterosexual marriage, all sexual activity outside of marriage must be immoral. This particular form of teleology was founded not only in theological belief about creation as mirroring God's purposes for humankind, but also in a Stoic philosophy of inherent purposes in nature.

Natural law formulations make up the heart of Roman Catholic teaching about sexual morality, excluding as gravely wrong not only homosexual acts, but masturbation, all marital acts carried out by contraceptive methods, and indeed, all sexual activity outside of matrimony. Whereas traditional natural law morality focused on the act as the centre of moral concern, recent developments in Rome have moved to a more Augustinian approach whereby the particular inclination of the homosexual person, though not itself a sin, is 'a more or less strong tendency ordered toward an intrinisic moral evil'.[9] This reflects a tendency to view sexual desire as itself evil.

One may note that the taboos against touching the genitals in Jewish and Christian tradition, and, in particular, the body of a person of the same sex, are distinctly a part of the religious culture that has formed the lives of millions of persons.[10]

The violation of the taboo is perceived by both society and the culprit as a world-destroying move, one that not only is dangerous but has immense erotic power resulting from a breaking of the boundaries between the familiar and the strange. That our society has set up the policing of toilets and the practice of police entrapment as part of its complex of social control only contributes to the walls of alienation that separate persons from one another. These taboos are clearly consequences of a natural law morality that becomes obsessed with control of sexual impulses and the need to channel libido into legitimized heterosexual arrangements where it will serve to further both reproduction and patriarchy.

Many modern Roman Catholic moral theologians have rejected this 'physiological teleology' in favor of a new morality of proportionalism and theories of compromise. In this way they have sought to avoid the 'naturalistic fallacy' whereby one arrived at moral obligations from the perceived ends of nature. Increasingly, they have recognized in the committed and stable homosexual union a good for those who have no alternative other than madness or a multitude of impersonal sexual contacts. Such thinking emerges from a contextual ethic that weighs goods and evils in terms of alternatives within the context of a person's possibilities. Exceptionless norms are put aside in favour of compromises that seek the greater good in a situation where absolutes cannot be realized. Few progressive moral theologians are ready to demand celibacy of persons who have no vocation or divinely conferred capacity for it. The moral theologian Daniel Maguire allows that a homosexual marriage may have internal validity within the framework of Catholic thought.[11]

André Guindon, a Canadian Catholic moral theologian, has argued extensively that a sexual ethic must not depend on the physical structure of an act 'according to nature' but on the truth or falsity of what it is saying to the person being embraced.[12] Guindon has argued against the notion that each physical organ has a purpose that excludes other purposes from being morally acceptable. He rejects the view that any human activity can be perfect, 'because it necessarily proceeds from an embodied, contextually situated, sexually differentiated and oriented, idiosyncratic, not fully actualized being'.[13] Guindon goes so far as to urge that 'homosexual acts of gays may receive a positive moral evaluation'.[14] This is because the fundamental self-evident maxim of Catholic moral theology is that one 'should act in accord with who one is (*agare sequitur esse*)'. In other words, one must not set up heterosexual norms for those who are not heterosexual.

Whereas in his earlier work Guindon rejected homosexuality as profoundly narcissistic, in his more recent work narcissism is regarded as only a pitfall to be overcome. For him the moral homosexual relationship is one in which the language of love is spoken by two persons who become an integrated couple. Their being of the same sex is basically irrelevant to the ethical character of the relationship. A similar stand on moral homosexual relations has been taken by the Protestant moral theologian James Nelson.[15] In addition, a 1979 report of the Church of England came down clearly in favour of bonded homosexual relations:

> In the light of some of the evidence we have received we do not think it possible to deny that there are circumstances in which individuals may justifiably choose to enter into a homosexual relationship with the hope of enjoying a companionship and physical expression of sexual love similar to that which is to be found in marriage. For the reasons which we have given such a relationship could not be regarded as the moral or social equivalent of marriage; it would be found to have a private and experimental character which marriage cannot and should not have. Nevertheless, fidelity and permanence, although not institutionally required, would undoubtedly do much to sustain and enhance its genuinely personal commitment and aspiration.[16]

A rather different approach is taken by Rabbi Hershel Matt, who upholds the traditional Jewish perspective that God's creation legitimizes and establishes heterosexuality as a norm for humanity. He goes on, however, to argue that the Halachic interpretation of Torah often recognized circumstances where freedom to adhere to the law was lacking (a principle known as *me ontes*).[17] The point here is not psychological freedom, but objective inability. Thus Israel was to obey the Sabbath regulations in obedience to God, but if the lives of Hebrew people were at stake, priority was to be given to defending those lives. Matt is aware that the Halachic authorities did not extend the concept of *me ontes* to homosexuals, but he believes that such extension would logically follow from what is now known about homosexuality. 'There seems to be', he states, 'near-unanimity: that for very many homosexuals the prospects of change to heterosexuality are almost nil.'[18]

The discussion of the Halachic status of homosexuality has become urgent and vociferous in Jewish circles. Robert Kirschner, for instance, has argued that Halakhah is not static and given once and for all.[19] According to this view, laws in the Halakhah do not follow from a priori ethical principles but from a posteriori conclusions drawn from Jewish experience. Thus although in the rabbinical tradition the deaf mute (*heresh*) was considered beyond all legal and moral responsibility because of his or her assumed imbecility, today we know that this assumption was not based on fact; hence the law must change. In the same way, we know that homosexuals are not heterosexuals who choose to act homosexually (as Torah assumed), but people whose orientation is definitively established in the deepest levels of their personality. Clearly, therefore, the assumption made in the Halakhah, where the context of idolatry and cultic prostitution was definitive for perverting a heterosexual person to homosexuality, does not apply.

Thus the rethinking of traditional Jewish and Christian attitudes towards homosexuality can assist members of the gay community in finding a moral way in which to live out their lives without conflict between their religion and their sexuality. Indeed, gays and lesbians have made much progress in spelling out an ethic for themselves. This ethic cannot, however, accept all the mores of the gay subculture. Specifically, it cannot accept the plurality of sexual partners that promoted the swift and devastating spread of AIDS. Insofar as all *nomos* was refused for homosexuals by the heterosexual community, of course, the anomie evident in the gay world was to some extent a consequence of that refusal;[20] if homosexuality was inherently evil, most gays had little alternative other than to live out a life without sexual norms. Nevertheless, with the advent of AIDS the free and easy lifestyle is gone forever. For those who wish to survive, it is a time for realism.

Those, however, who had little use for straight sexual morality before AIDS may have little use for it now. Indeed, a leading gay advocate, Dennis Altman, has reaffirmed his belief that 'gay relationships are not based upon an assumption of monogamy.'[21] In his later work he persists in thinking that this is beyond the ability of gays and affirms that the de-emphasization of sexual satisfaction and the substitution of solitary masturbation provide the only realistic alternative for gay men.[22] Prior to the emergence of AIDS, gay liberation was often conceived of as freedom from all restraints imposed by a hostile heterosexual milieu. Overcoming self-hatred (often the legacy of incorporating negative attitudes of the homophobic straight community) was a first priority in learning to love and respect oneself.

Thus refusal to submit to the expectations of a dominant society that in the past has offered little more than persecution is understandable; there is a parallel with the women's movement in many gays' insistence that it is they who must take control of their lives.

But the situation today has clearly changed, and other gay men find this a time for creating stable and faithful sexual relationships of mutual commitment. Though one cannot base a morality of sexual relations solely upon the pragmatic grounds of health and safety, any way of reducing the number of sexual partners and changing sexual practices to avoid exchanges of body fluids (a change evident in some data recently collected from San Francisco, for example) is beneficial.[23]

The translation of the principle of 'do no harm' into the obligation of safer sex is fundamental in a sexual ethic. No sexual act can be moral that is left open to the possibility of HIV infection. Thus it is essential that the morality of condom use be affirmed over against the official position of the Vatican.[24] There is much evidence, however, that condoms fail in at least ten per cent of usage.[25] Therefore we must speak of 'safer sex' with condoms rather than 'safe sex'.

In the light of these dangers, the limitation of sexual activity to bonded couples who are HIV-negative makes the creation of homosexual marriages something that is both socially and morally desirable. This is so not only for pragmatic reasons but also because of the values of commitment and personal relatedness that make sexuality more human. In his understanding of sexuality as a language, Guindon has shown how vital love – heterosexual or homosexual – is to the well-being of committed partners. The use of a paradigm of communicative sharing as a form of fecundity takes us beyond the teleological concerns of the Vatican hierarchy and their negative attitudes towards all homosexual expression. It is also important, however, to spell out what values are to be realized in the moral homosexual relationship.

It is not at all self-evident that monogamy as it has existed for heterosexual marriages is what gays and lesbians should aim at in their sexual arrangements. Monogamy is embedded in an ideology built on possession and property as guiding norms within marriage. Non-monogamy, on the other hand, is not necessarily the answer, since it is only a negation of monogamy that leaves the primary relationship so open to invasion from the outside that it can hardly be said to exist. Some gays, pointing to differences between affirmational and recreational sex, have found the two compatible with one another.[26] In this view, bonding involves a combination of the two so as to protect the primary relationship and raise it to a high level of personal commitment, even if that commitment is not necessarily life-long.

Only those who realize the essential ambiguity of sexual identity can provide the compassionate acceptance of homosexual persons with AIDS that is required of those providing care. This is put very well by Dr Stuart Nichols:

> If human sexuality is thought of as being a continuum between heterosexuality and homosexuality in everyone, many of these problems would be minimized or eliminated. The sense of a basic difference between gay and nongay people would be removed, as would the imaginary danger now attached to the recognition of one's intrinsic homoerotic feeling.[27]

In the absence of such understanding, however, homosexuality remains the mirror in which 'normal' persons look to see what they must not be. The opposition of weak versus strong, evil versus good, feminine versus masculine, always puts the gay or lesbian person in an unfavourable category. The accusation that gays are effeminate only reveals a latent hatred for the feminine itself as that which real men must avoid in themselves.[28]

So also the 'masculine woman' is scorned since she implies a fundamental threat to the man who exalts his masculinity. Keeping oneself free of any emotional or erotic ties to persons of the same sex is a way of maintaining an intrinsically fragile gender identity. The belief that gender categories are intrinsic qualities rather than constructs serving purposes including domination and social control is one that dies with difficulty.[29]

Indeed, the enforcement of gender boundaries is part of the conspiracy by which patriarchy extends and defends itself. Even the celibate elite of the Roman Catholic Church are pledged to the support of the patriarchal system through their natural law ethic and its enforcement in the Church by use of the confessional. This is why homosexuality is viewed as such a perverse and evil phenomenon by the Catholic hierarchy – and all the more so as it remains an ever-present temptation for those who have rejected heterosexual marriage in favor of celibacy. Those who embrace a homosexual lifestyle are punished and excluded from a community that at the same time values the qualities of such persons. Gays and lesbians are considered to be traitors to the cause and, indeed, moral heretics.[30]

The fact that relatively few Christians have been ready to stand up and support gay and lesbian people since the advent of AIDS indicates that sexual heretics are still fair game for inquisitions.[31] If the religious communities cannot do without the category of 'the heretic' it is imperative that they grasp the absolute prohibition of destroying other human beings in the name of God or of blessing an epidemic that is invoked as God's will for sinners. Religious maturity demands that our orthodoxies not be furthered by morally blaming the heretics. At the very least the churches should recognize that the 'sin' of homosexuality, if it be such, is involuntary.

The Jewish and Christian traditions have recognized a degree of self-autonomy in the legitimacy of conscience. Those Catholic gay men who insist on remaining in the Church despite the attempts of Vatican officials to turn them out do so in the name of conscience, remaining loyal to their partners in the name of Christ and living in covenants of mutual care and love without the blessing of the Church. Brian McNaught has gone so far as to argue that in another generation these Catholic gay men will be seen as the equivalents of martyrs like Joan of Arc, who stood up to the Church that burned her.[32] In the American Episcopalian Church, the Bishop of Newark, John Spong, has suggested that a liturgical blessing for same-sex marriages be established,[33] and various bishops are ready to approve such a move. Indeed, he already has one for use in his diocese.

Granting greater freedoms to homosexual people to make their own moral decisions according to their conscience does not detract from the validity of heterosexual marriage as a state of life blessed by the church or synagogue. There are simply different vocations, as the callings to monastic life and marriage have been recognized to be within Catholicism. It is entirely possible that the attempt on the part of many gays to seek out stable, long-term relationships of fidelity under the life-threatening conditions created by the AIDS epidemic can be linked with the move on the part of many Jews and Christians to be more open to the goodness of those gay and lesbian relationships that mirror love, fidelity, and commitment. Simon Watney has argued that this conservative move against the 'promiscuity' that is often named as a contributing factor in the AIDS epidemic is only the re-emergence of a religious ethic, at heart opposed to gay life.[34] I, on the other hand, would interpret AIDS as an indicator that multiple sexual partners are risky not only to health but to the quality of relationship that is a mark of what it is to be more fully human and mature.

It has been the task of this essay to present an alternative religious reading of the AIDS epidemic to that presented by homophobic and punitive reactions to AIDS. Just as the equation of AIDS with punishment came from the equation of homosexual activity with sin, so if we free homosexuality from the stigma of being contrary to nature or the will of God, an alternative reading can interpret AIDS as a condition calling forth compassion and care. The acceptance of responsible homosexual relations as having equal authenticity with heterosexual relations can rescue us from the condemnation of gay persons as sinners. Only by changing negative attitudes can we overcome the stigmatization of PWAs that many of us find so abhorrent. We must, as the Second Vatican Council insisted, read the signs of the times. In the time of the holocaust of the Jews, anti-Semitism had to be banished forever. In the time of the pandemic of AIDS, so also must homophobia be banished from our communities. Only then can homosexuals accept their condition as a particular vocation to be realized in love, fidelity, and responsibility to the significant other to whom one is called.

NOTES

[1] Quoted in Mary E. Hunt, 'An Invitation to Rethink Sexuality: A Christian Feminist Liberation Perspective', in David G. Hallman, ed., *AIDS Issues: Confronting the Challenge* (New York: Pilgrim Press, 1989), p. 214.

[2] Ibid.

[3] The most obvious example of this approach is *The AIDS Coverup?* by Gene Antonio. Such scare tactics and militant homophobia would place this book in the wastebasket prepared for the work of cranks if it were not that the book has sold over 200,000 copies since 1986 and was published by the Ignatius Press, a Catholic firm that also publishes such reputable theological works as those of Hans Urs von Balthasar.

[4] Stuart Nichols, 'The Social Climate When AIDS Developed', in David G. Ostrow, ed., *The Psychiatric Implications of the Acquired Immune Deficiency Syndrome* (Washington, DC: American Psychiatric Press, 1984), p. 91.

[5] René Girard, *The Scapegoat* (Baltimore, MD: Johns Hopkins University Press, 1988).

[6] Susan Sontag, *Illness as Metaphor* (New York: Farrar, Straus, Giroux, 1977). Sontag reiterates her approach in *AIDS and Its Metaphors* (New York: Farrar, Straus, Giroux, 1989).

[7] This seems to be the position of Andrew Halloran in his book *Ground Zero* (New York: New American Library, 1988), pp. 17–18.

[8] Hershel Matt, 'Sin, Crime, Sickness or Alternative Life Style: A Jewish Approach to Homosexuality', in Edward Batchelor, ed., *Homosexuality and Ethics* (New York: Pilgrim Press, 1980), p. 118.

[9] Sacred Congregation for the Doctrine of the Faith, 'Letter to the Bishops of the Catholic Church on the Pastoral Care of Homosexual Persons' 3, in Jeannine Gramick and Pat Furey, eds, *The Vatican and Homosexuality* (New York: Crossroad, 1988), p. 2.

[10] The Talmud is firm in prohibiting boys from touching their penis during urination since it leads to masturbation, which is strongly tabooed. Similar prohibitions are evident in traditional Catholic moral theology, where touching one's own 'indecent parts' or those of another without a reasonable cause is designated as sinful. Heribert Jones and Urban Adelman, *Moral Theology* (Westminster, MD: Newman Press, 1953) pp. 154–5.

[11] Daniel Maguire, 'The Morality of Homosexual Marriage', in Robert Nugent, ed., *A Challenge to Love: Gay and Lesbian Catholics in the Church* (New York: Crossroad, 1983).

[12]André Guindon, *The Sexual Creators: An Ethical Proposal for Concerned Christians* (Landon, MD: University Press of America, 1986), pp. 159-204.

[13]Ibid., p. 161.

[14]Ibid.

[15]James B. Nelson, 'Religious and Moral Issues in Working with Homosexual Clients', in John C. Gonsiorek, ed., *A Guide to Psychotherapy with Gay and Lesbian Clients* (New York: Harrington Park Press, 1985).

[16]*Homosexual Relationships* (London: Church of England Board of Social Responsibility, 1979), p. 52.

[17]Matt, p. 17.

[18]Ibid., pp. 118-19.

[19]Robert Kirschner, 'Halakhah and Homosexuality: A Reappraisal', *Judaism* 37 (Fall 1988): 450-8.

[20]The immoral and anomic aspects of the gay ghetto have been chronicled by many authors, but the most articulate statement has been made by Marshall Kirk and Hunter Madsen in their book *After the Ball: How America Will Conquer Its Fear and Hatred of Gays in the 90s* (New York: Doubleday, 1989). The entire book is a call to responsibility and bonded relationships as the only way to the acceptance of gays by the straight community and the avoidance of a potential holocaust of homosexuals in the aftermath of the AIDS crisis. Many critics within the gay world have reacted with nothing short of contempt for the proposals of Kirk and Madsen.

[21]Dennis Altman, *The Homosexualization of America* (New York: St Martin's Press, 1982), p. 175.

[22]Dennis Altman, *AIDS in the Mind of America* (Garden City, NY: Anchor Press/ Doubleday, 1986), pp. 158-9.

[23]Diane Johnson and John F. Murray, 'AIDS without End', *New York Review of Books* 35, 13 (18 Aug. 1988): 59. The reference is to the Presentation at the Twentieth Annual Meeting of the Society for Epidemiological Research, University of California, San Francisco (17 June 1987) made by N.A. Hessol *et al.*

[24]The American Catholic hierarchy has been split over the legitimate use of and education about condom use. The Catholic moral theologian John Tuohey has written a persuasive article in favor of the morality of condom use to avoid HIV infection, though without addressing homosexual use of condoms ('Methodology or Ideology: The Condom and a Consistent Sexual Ethic', *Louvain Studies* 25, 1 (1990): 53-69).

[25]Helen Kaplan, 'AIDS and the Sex Therapist', editorial, *Sex and Marital Therapy* 11, 4 (Winter 1985): 210-14, and J.J. Goldert, 'What Is Safe Sex?', *New England Journal of Medicine* 257 (January 1987): 640-4.

[26]Perhaps the best account is in the little classic of Don Clark, *Loving Someone Gay* (New York: New American Library, 1977).

[27]Nichols, p. 90.

[28]This is stated very clearly by Richard Isay in his book *Being Homosexual: Gay Men and Their Development* (New York: Farrar, Straus, Giroux, 1989), p. 78.

[29]Michael Kaufman, 'The Construction of Masculinity and the Triad of Men's Violence', in Michael Kaufman, ed., *Beyond Patriarchy: Essays by Men on Pleasure, Power, and Changes* (Toronto: Oxford University Press, 1987), pp. 1-29.

[30]Ivan Illich identifies the link between doctrinal heresy and homosexuality as moral heresy in his book *Gender* (New York: Pantheon, 1982), p. 149.

[31]Timothy C. Potts has exposed the activities of the Roman Sacred Congregation for the Doctrine of the Faith in his article 'Joseph Ratzinger and the New Inquisition', in *The European Gay Review* 2: 90-104.

[32]Brian McNaught, *On Being Gay* (New York: St Martin, 1988).

[33]John S. Spong, *Living in Sin* (San Francisco: Harper & Row, 1988).

[34]Simon Watney, *Policing Desire: Pornography, AIDS, and the Media* (Minneapolis: University of Minnesota Press, 1987).

ACQUIRED IMMANENT DIVINITY SYNDROME

JAMES MILLER

No single term in official AIDS discourse has done more damage to the morale of people with HIV disease, or provoked more debate over the ethics of representation in the politically charged field of AIDS awareness, than the dooming label 'victim'. What I shall criticize in this essay is not the label itself – which is only a word – but the translation of its shifting meanings into a fixed identity for the people on whom it is now, fairly casually, imposed.

I think it quite wrong to maintain, though it has been fervently argued, that people with AIDS (PWAs) should never be regarded or described as victims, for many of them have surely been victimized and even vanquished by hostile forces ranging from pathogens to politicians. To deny their profound experience of loss and defeat is to misunderstand their own dauntless point that they are 'living with AIDS' despite the gloom and doom broadcast by the mainstream media. My critical intention, rather, is to consider why PWAs have so often been burdened with this label, and how their public identity as victims of various sorts (guilty, innocent, disenfranchised, sacrificial) works both for and against them in their valiant efforts to assert their rights as 'persons' in the face of depersonalizing government agendas and dehumanizing social attitudes.

Starting from the basic Foucauldian assumption that representation is an essentially political process, I shall explore in the first section of this essay the complex implications of the victim label vis-à-vis the presumed guilt or innocence of the infected. Then, in the second section, I shall consider the growing popularity of a religious variant of the victim role – namely, the PWA as martyr – in relation to conservative political doctrines and the countercultural ethos of AIDS activism. In the final section, a critical reading of the first full-blown AIDS saint's life, I shall conclude with some reflections on the need for PWAs and their allies to resist the cultural imposition of any nomenclature that sets them apart from the general public.

My argument *against* isolationist representations (i.e., images of PWAs that figuratively quarantine their experiences from those of the general public) will necessarily concern invisible things like value systems, political structures, apocalyptic fears, and immortal longings. To ground my discussion in the visible world, I have constructed my argument *for* inclusionary representations (those that promote socially constructive interactions between the sick and the well) by drawing attention to several actual images of PWAs as martyrs drawn from the media, the fine arts, and the non-medical literature of AIDS.

THE VICTIM DEBATE

Despite the concerted efforts of activist artists and critics to eliminate the 'victim' label from all discussions of the epidemic, it is still firmly lodged in what media commentators (appearing not to refer to themselves) like to call 'the Popular Mind'. Anyone seeking a way into the world of the Popular Mind should scan the headlines of the tabloid press.

'AIDS VICTIMS CAGED FOR BIZARRE EXPERIMENTS', shrieked the front page of the 30 January 1990 issue of the *Weekly World News*, a tabloid sold in supermarkets throughout Canada and the United States. This revelation (prefaced with 'Top secret report rocks the medical world!') hooked me into turning to page five, where my worst fears about the World were confirmed: 'AIDS VICTIMS TURNED INTO HUMAN GUINEA PIGS!'

To prove this claim, the *Weekly World News* printed a photograph of a fat black-gowned nurse drawing blood from the veins of a black man who had poked his arm through a small round hole (see Figure 1). Here, it seemed, was the anus of the medical world, the dangerous convergence point of desire and death for seropositive gays caught in the infamous act of 'fisting' by the offended patriarchy. Here, in the secret theatre of anal torments, the medical gaze has become a voyeuristic stare fixing its sorry victims in parodic tableaux of deviant sexuality to titillate all who read the *Weekly World News* religiously.[1]

Is there any other way to read such strong stuff? Tabloids are the martyrologies of the Popular Mind. The 'AIDS victims' in the photo have been sacrificed to a moralized system of repressive political values normally hidden from the mass audience by the clouds of divinized Hierarchical Authority. But here, like a flash of mystical insight, the photo reveals the apocalyptic truth behind the scenes – the heartless workings of the World, the ghastly captivity of the Flesh, the relentless cruelties of the Devil. This is all dished out as eschatological evidence confirming the 'top-secret report', which of course 'rocks the medical world' because it is essentially a religious revelation.

'Hellish hospital is located in the eastern part of Cuba', reads the caption beneath an insert box providing a helpful map of the Devil's new Caribbean headquarters (Figure 2). The very name of the site, Los Cocos, sounds fiendishly homoerotic.

Martyrs traditionally see their heavenly crowns descending long before they feel them on their heads. At once divine and human, their peculiar perspective on life is curiously evoked in the *Weekly World News*: while the visionary photo of the 'AIDS victims' reveals the government of the World in all its horror from the judgemental viewpoint of God, the story beneath it plunges the reader into the *de profundis* horrors of the earthly victims. When they are not being 'drained of their blood, pumped full of experimental drugs and operated on without anaesthesia', they are 'locked away and forced to live like lepers in grim stainless steel and glass cells'. Their imposed isolation is a *reductio ad horrorem* of the fundamentalist fantasy of AIDS as the ultimate alienation of the soul from God and the Good Society.

Yet the reporter, Beatrice Dexter, surprisingly does not damn the caged deviants for their manifold sins and wickedness, but does everything in her limited rhetorical power to redeem them in the eyes and hearts of her readers. In her report the McCarthyite discourse of Democracy as the moral opposite of Communism is so strong that it not only overpowers but miraculously reverses the usual right-wing tendency to represent seropositive queers and junkies as guilty AIDS victims, sinners who asked for God's judgement and got it in viral form. Before our very eyes they are translated into martyrs for Democracy.

Their ascetic separation from the World is ironically confirmed by the God's-eye glimpse of their cells in the photo, a still, surely, from Foucault's worst nightmare of population control through categorical individuation and totalitarian hospital management. 'Let's face it,' chortles a Government Bigwig quoted in a box over the captive patients, 'these are drug addicts and homosexuals who are going to die anyway.' Let's face it indeed: not the Grand Guignol fantasy of a living morgue (a stock image in the apocalyptic tabloids) but the old fascist agenda of quarantine and extermination, which is seriously proposed from time to time by perfectly respectable AIDS commentators who wouldn't be caught dead reading the *Weekly World News*.[2]

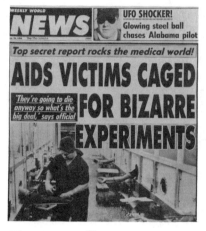

FIGURE 1, *see* page 56.

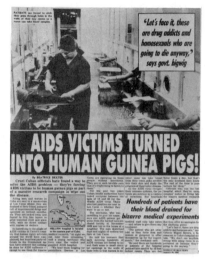

FIGURE 2, *see* page 57.

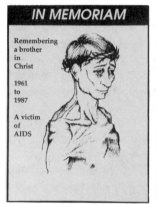

FIGURE 3, *see* page 63.

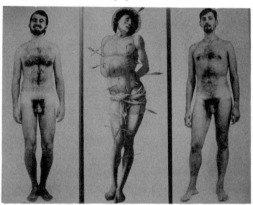

FIGURE 4, *see* page 64.

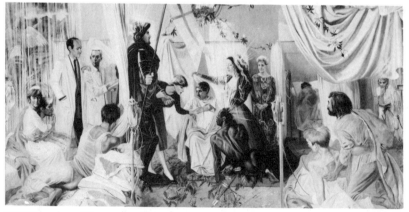

FIGURE 5, *see* page 65.

Dexter's report, trashy as it is, should be taken seriously as a sign of the increasingly popular displacement of a McCarthyite AIDS discourse (and the isolationist agenda that goes with it) away from America as its field of reference onto a traditional site of American political angst and frustration. Why this displacement? I suspect it reflects a collective wish: the Popular Mind, wishing 'to wipe out the disease' (yet frustrated by the failure of Medical Science) finds it easy to imagine the old political alternative – wiping out the diseased – occurring in a distant communist hell-hole, but altogether too hard to face it happening right here at home. Yet who can doubt that somewhere in the 'Free World' at this very moment people with AIDS are getting the plastic-glove treatment from hostile hospital staff, or are being pumped full of experimental drugs for the sake of medical research, or are forced to live like lepers in grim stainless-steel and glass cells?

Media representations of 'AIDS victims' need not be as sensational as the images in the *Weekly World News* to have the same isolationist effect: recent mainstream press coverage of the epidemic of pediatric AIDS in Romania encourages a similar complacent belief in the general public that the AIDS Crisis at its victimizing worst is really happening far, far away, to innocent foreigners caught in corrupt medical systems, even though seropositive men and women in the Free World are desperately volunteering for guinea-pig duty in underground drug trials because conservative governments are loath to reliquish control over the protocols of medicine.

Radical voices have been raised for some time now against the dual discourse of conservative judgementalism and biomedical objectification underlying the representation of AIDS patients as guilty or innocent victims conveniently separable from the rest of humanity. 'We condemn attempts to label us as "victims", which implies defeat,' proclaimed the founders of the People with AIDS Coalition in 1985, 'and we are only occasionally "patients", which implies passivity, helplessness, and dependence upon the care of others.' Echoing the gender-neutral idiom of American feminism and the defiantly proud tone of Gay Liberation, these undoomable rebels went on to assert their democratic right to represent themselves by a bold act of communal naming: 'We are "people with AIDS".'[3] As authors of their own name, PWAs have asserted an authority over their destinies and become impatient activists in the tradition of the Civil Rights Movement.

Unfortunately, not all people with AIDS have what it takes to be People With AIDS. Someone may have the minimal requirement, HIV disease, with none of the other essential PWA qualifications – faith in the democratic process, commitment to activist aesthetic practices, loads of political energy, gay-positivity, community spirit, guts, and hope. Perhaps a great many people with AIDS simply have no place in the heroic activist picture, because the picture itself, as an idealistic vision of social and sexual liberation, tends to gloss over the harsh realities of their weakened physical state. It pressures them to be what they may not or cannot be, social paragons, at a time when society is willy-nilly turning them into pariahs. It may even make them feel guilty for not living up to the high ideal of Living With AIDS.

'Under the rules of AIDSpeak,' argued journalist Randy Shilts in an Orwellian analysis of official AIDS discourse, 'AIDS victims could never be called victims. Instead they were to be called People With AIDS, or PWAs, as if contracting this uniquely brutal disease was not a victimizing experience.'[4] Contracting the terms of the disease was an insult heaped upon the injury of contracting the disease itself, he insisted, because the 'euphemistic' character of AIDSpeak promoted complacency in the general public (and in govern-ment bureaucracies) rather than liberal sympathy or activist outrage. Ironi-cally, to the people with AIDS who invented the abbreviations Shilts disparages, AIDSpeak was anything but euphemistic. It was self-empowering. The gay political leaders and public-health officials who bor-rowed the term 'PWA' from PWA Coalition founder Michael Callen did so out of respect for the political agenda of the very people who were most actively protesting the 'victimizing experience' of media misrepresentation.[5]

Shilts's call-a-victim-a-victim argument ties together the many AIDS patient biographies narrated in his Dickensian chronicle *And the Band Played On: Politics, People, and the AIDS Epidemic*. In the harrowing tale of Gary Walsh, for instance, Shilts pushes the victim role to new heights by describing the public apotheosis of a 'typical' plague-victim into a healing saint. Walsh, a San Francisco therapist, was diagnosed with AIDS in 1983, and in the year following his diagnosis lesbian activist Lu Chaikin watched adversity trans-form her friend by stripping away the pretensions of personality 'layer by layer, until [his] altruistic essence was all that remained'.[6] No diet prescribed by the Church Fathers could have a more ascetic effect on Gary than the Gay Plague, which even succeeded in erasing from his memory 'the hurts of his Catholic childhood and the abuses he had suffered as a gay man'. Now that he offered his friends 'unconditional love', people came away from conversa-tions with Gary 'like pilgrims leaving a holy shrine'.

As an AIDS victim, Gary will outgrow the traditionally second-rate Cath-olic role of the *martyrus in spiritu* (martyr in spirit): the unspecified hurts of his pre-AIDS life will appear as nothing compared with the transfiguring tor-ments of the disease. These offer him an opportunity to become a first-rate witness to the therapeutic glories of Love Triumphant, a true *martyrus in corpore* (which was the privileged role for an early Christian because it entailed death in the arena). It is an opportunity he gladly takes. Dispatching his pilgrims with a zap of unconditional love, he finds the strength to exclaim to Lu before snuffing out his little candle in the darkness of the Flesh: 'I got it, I finally got it! . . . I *am* love and light, and I transform people by just being who I am.'

Just what did he get in the end? A hagiographical mutation of AIDS that we can only diagnose from its luminous symptoms as Acquired Immanent

Divinity Syndrome. Lu, of course, 'broke down and started weeping' because she 'felt that a flame had been passed'. Gary's Christ-like participation in the 'altruistic essence' of the Godhead has transformed her into a weeping Magdalen. The flame passed to her was none other than the Holy Spirit blazing off the Divine Presence immanent in Human Form, and like the disciples at Pentecost she must now pass on the flame to the journalists waiting at the hospital door.

The pop-cult martyrology of the redeemable and transfigurable AIDS victim, that staple of the tabloid press, depends upon constant mainstream articulation of a full-blown AIDS Apocalypse by mediating 'experts' like Shilts who have risen above the *Weekly World News*. 'AIDS is evidently still such an embarrassing subject for most journalists that they will stop at nothing to compass and confine the experience of people with AIDS in their own insultingly victimising terms,' observed British gay activist Simon Watney in 1987: 'That is why we must refuse, absolutely, to inhabit the immensely convenient role of the "victim", which has been so generously dug to contain us like a mass grave.'[7]

Where Shilts saw the role of the AIDS victim as an ascetic route to immortality, Watney presents it as a dead end – the site of mass murder – by evoking the genocidal horror of the Nazi era. Breaking the silence that equals death, he urges all gay people to oppose the tragic discourse of the AIDS crisis and to replace the lives of the saints with the Nuremburg Trial records as the best model for the AIDS narrative. 'We know that if our species has any worth or beauty, it lies in its diversity, and our capacity to embrace and celebrate all our variously consenting states of desire,' he preaches at the end of *Policing Desire*: 'And if in these terrible times we should wish somewhat to alleviate the pain of our losses – of freedoms and of friends – then we might think of AIDS as a monstrously ironic means to this end, and of our loved ones who have died as martyrs to that great cause.'[8]

An unexpected revision of the terms in the victim debate may be noted here. Instead of deconstructing the language of tabloid Toryism, Watney faces the silent legions of the AIDS dead so that their widely ignored deaths will have some meaning in relation to a cause greater (for him) than PWA rights – the survival of Gay Liberation, under whose now ragged banner of Sexual Diversity they are enlisted as 'martyrs' in a fully religious sense, with no trace of irony.

Thus reinvented by Watney, the multitude lost to HIV march forward as the Protectors of Diversity against the Policers of Desire. Martyrs may look like passive victims to the cynical spectator, but to the true believer whose eyes are shocked open by pain, those who die for the Great Cause (however defined) offer consolation to the living as the ultimate activists, the eternal victors.

THREE SYMPTOMS OF IMMANENT DIVINITY

We have now seen martyrs crowned on both sides of the victim debate, though for opposing reasons. On the one hand, mainstream journalists who argue for the victim label present the martyrdom of gay PWAs (who are never quite the 'innocent victims' that seropositive babies or the wives of closeted bisexuals are) as a miraculous transcendence of worldly evil. On the other hand, PWAs and their allies tend to appropriate the dead to their justly furious but fracturing resistance movement and proclaim them martyrs to this or that unifying cause for social change, be it Gay Liberation or Women's Rights or what you will.

The radicals even act out the public drama of martyrdom as an arena massacre followed by a mass resurrection in a brilliantly ironic ritual known as a 'Die-In'. In this parody of a hippie 'Love-In', volunteers fall 'dead' on the sidewalk and limply hold tombstone-shaped placards over their bodies protesting this or that government outrage while their comrades chant the credo of ACT UP: 'Not Victims! Not Patients! But People Living With AIDS!' Then, at a signal from their leader, the dead rise from their temporary graves to join the living in their war against the imperialistic Establishment. Their martyr's insignia, the Pink Triangle, is an inverted form of the badge sewn onto the uniforms of homosexual prisoners in the Nazi concentration camps. AIDS is clearly presented as their Holocaust, and they are its sacrificial victims.[9]

Strictly speaking, of course, the Church (at least its Catholic branch) cannot canonize a martyred PWA or even consider such a person martyred simply because he or she died of AIDS. The crown of martyrdom is awarded by God and recognized by His official servants only when three conditions are met by the candidate. First, the person must really have died. Suffering in itself is not enough to transform a life of pain into Light and Love or to justify a sufferer in the technical sense of wiping away all spots of sin from the soul. Second, the person's death must be inflicted as a murder by a sinner or group of sinners acting out of hatred for Christian doctrine or virtue. This condition rules out all deaths by 'natural causes' as well as fatal accidents and mercy killings. The third condition is perhaps the most important: the prospective martyr must have voluntarily accepted death in defence of Christian doctrine or virtue.[10]

Suppose that a Catholic PWA fulfilled the first two conditions of martyrdom by dying at the hands of wicked oppressors who despised his patience under adversity. Only by willing his death in some sense – without committing suicide – could he turn victim into victor and satisfy the third condition of martyrdom. Now suppose that he volunteered for hellish experimental drug treatments (unlike the Los Cocos victims) and survived them long enough to become a celebrated AIDS activist for, say, HIV-positive prisoners. If he bravely refused all further treatments and went on a hunger strike to draw world attention to the plight of PWAs in the prison system, his claim to a martyr's crown would be fairly strong – unless, of course, he was gay: the merest hint of sexual 'perversion' would disqualify him as a martyr in the eyes of the Catholic Church as currently constituted.

Winning a crimson crown might still be possible for gay PWAs, however, if they joined the Anglican Church. So we might infer from the October 1987 issue of *The Anglican Magazine*, which featured a complementary pair of articles on a young 'brother in Christ' who was also a 'victim of AIDS'. The first article ('Living with AIDS, and Death: WHAT AM I?') is an identity–crisis essay by the victim himself, who is simply identified as 'David'. Though editor John Bird piously affixes the 'victim' label to his subject, David himself rejects it in his personal manifesto of moral victory over the churchy types who would disapprove of his gayness and prefer to see him as a victim of *it*. 'I am the the boy next door,' he proudly proclaims, 'I am your brother. I am not a victim.'[11] Maybe not, but as Bird notes, David died at the age of 25 after serving in the Anglican Youth Movement. Whether there is a causal connection between these two biographical facts we are left to wonder as we turn to the second article, which turns out to be a morally edifying *legendum* of David's martyrdom written by his mother, who naturally 'could never have made it through this without faith'.[12]

Also faithful to martyrological tradition is the illustration that precedes these articles. Sandra Peplar's (see Figure 3) image of a skinny, prematurely aged, gay white male wearing a crown of thorns is a masterpiece of pious overstatement, just the sort of hyperbole needed to turn a good Anglican Youth into a Christ-figure. *Ecce Homo*: here is the gay Man of Sorrows who has evidently made it as a Soldier of the Cross through the old route of *imitatio Christi*.

Christ is identified in Revelation 1:5 as 'the faithful witness', an epithet referring either to his divine wisdom as the seer who penetrates God's Mysteries, or to his full and voluntary experience of mortality as 'the first-born of the dead' to rise into glory. Because of this epithet, the early Church tended to promote the popular veneration of Christ as the prototypical martyr in a historical sense – that is, the first victim of anti-Christian persecution.

Perhaps Revelation was in the artist's mind when she drew the crucified Arch-Martyr as the prototypical PWA. It would certainly come as a revelation to most PWAs that AIDS is the gay man's path to glory as an imitation of Christ's suffering and death. The physical torment of the syndrome and the social humiliations attending it are David's crucifixion, which not only tests but proves his superhuman fortitude (the virtue traditionally associated with the martyrs). Through a brave sacrifice of his youth, his looks, his health, and his worldly future, he has acquired something other-worldly as a clone of Christ. Look into his over-sized eyes, and behold the glow of mystical wisdom: the first symptom of immanent divinity.

The second symptom is a radiant corporeal integrity that results from restoration of the martyr's broken body through the healing grace of the First Martyr in his heavenly role as Christ the Victor. The martyrs in Michelangelo's *Last Judgement* stand up, or float up, on heroically reformed bodies, presumably the 'spiritual bodies' that, according to St Paul (I Cor. 15:44), shall rise where their carnal bodies were sown on the worldly battlefield. A Before-and-After contrast is always implicit in such scenes. Normally it is suggested by the presentation in the martyrs' hands of the very instruments of torture that broke their bodies but not their spirits in the arena of this Life. Catherine presents her wheel, and Lawrence his grill, and Sebastian his arrows as if their celestial show-and-tell proved the invulnerability of their glorified bodies to such inglorious weapons of persecution. Occasionally, as in Michelangelo's portrait of St Bartholomew, the apocalyptic contrast between Before and After is marked by a brutally simple juxtaposition of the Flesh Incorruptible with the ripped, bloodied, shredded, punctured, roasted, or flayed skin of the martyr's fallen body. No instruments of torture need then be presented to the viewer. The Flesh says it all.[13]

Wishing for physical wholeness is something most of us do when we're sick, but fulfilling that wish as a sign of spiritual triumph over the Flesh is something only martyrs have traditionally enjoyed. Now PWAs can do it too if they acquire immanent divinity through artistic intercession. Two PWAs who have recently acquired it – much to their surprise, no doubt, since at the time they posed for their portraits neither knew he was infected with HIV – stand up like proud sentinels to display their woundless bodies on either side of St Sebastian in a defiantly candid triptych by Canadian artist David Horsley (see Figure 4).

Horsley's Sebastian, copied from Mantegna's celebrated portrait of the early Roman martyr, is still suffering in the Flesh, his pierced and twisted body contrasting sharply with the vertical at-ease stances of the victorious outer figures. The contrast between tortured and triumphant bodies is further marked by the presentation of the semi-nude Sebastian in acrylic flesh tones and his fully naked avatars in black and white silver prints on a fluorescent white background. Now, thanks to AIDS, Sebastian, whose bound figure has been subversively eroticized and idolized by generations of gay men, is to be viewed again as an interceding martyr for the plague-stricken, which is his traditional Catholic role.[14]

Talismanic images, such as the St Sebastian banners paraded through Renaissance towns during outbreaks of the Plague, are designed to influence rather than simply reflect the life-struggles of the sick. Horsley himself does not go so far as to claim talismanic virtues for his plague icon. But it's a short step from his discovery of the oracular potency of martyr imagery to the magical breakthrough into the wholly iconic world of curative talismans, where the third and ultimate symptom of immanent divinity – the acquisition of miraculous healing powers – is revealed and demonstrated to the venerators of a dead PWA. To enter this world, we have to make more than a leap of faith. We have to vault over the drab wards of mundane reason and check into the top floor of the Hospital of the Mysteries.

The elevator of mystical fantasy has been taken all the way to the top by the British-based Canadian painter André Durand in 'Votive Offering', a massive Renaissance-style altarpiece, also in triptych form, completed in 1987 (see Figure 5). Here, in the strange glow of saintly aureoles, we can make out a hospital ward such as few PWAs are likely to see without the aid of hallucinatory drugs to focus their inner eye on the martyrological miracle occurring in the centre.

The central panel depicts the rebirth of Sunnye Sherman, an American PWA who died in 1986.[15] Her visionary renaissance is attended by that media-hallowed AIDS activist, Princess Diana, along with a trio of healing saints. As the Straight Woman of Sorrows undone by the viral sperm of a bisexual tormentor, Sunnye rises again in 'Votive Offering' with all the symptoms of immanent divinity. Her eyes glow with supernal wisdom as if the shaft of Divine Light streaming through the celestial roundel over her head had possessed her soul and driven away the darkness of AIDS dementia. Her body, once so frail that sitting up in bed had been a major undertaking, now sits as tall as Duccio's 'Virgin in Majesty'.

To mystical vision and corporeal integrity we can now add the third blessing: a glamorous revirginalization that heals all who behold its glory. Like the white robes of the Brides of Christ, Sunnye's nightgown betokens her immaculate reconception as a virgin saint whose transcendence of suffering does not take her away from the world but rather brings her back into play, body and spirit, with those who still suffer as she did the arrow-wounds of the Plague. Healed by the magical synapse of Diana's Royal Touch, Sunnye can now function in her own right as a victorious healing force in the realm of the Living Dead.

With all this celestial therapy going on at the centre, no wonder the male AIDS patients in the outer panels of the triptych are craning their necks and lifting their sick brethren to catch a glimpse of Our Lady of AIDS. They want a divine zap too – a touch from the cool hand of the thaumaturgical princess, a ray from Sebastian's halo, a smile from triumphant Sunnye. Anything.

Why has Durand imaginatively translated Sunnye's remains from the American hospital where she died to a British Monarchist shrine? Perhaps for the same essentially political reasons that early Christian bishops had the relics of celebrity martyrs literally 'translated' or 'carried across' from the usually pagan site of martyrdom to a sanctified locus where miracles could officially occur under clerical supervision. In the healing shrine or 'martyrium', the eternal glory of the saints could redound solely on the local commander of the Church Militant and beef up the temporal prestige of the Ecclesiastical Hierarchy.[16]

By transforming a gloomy AIDS ward into a martyrium blooming with vitalistic passion-flowers, Durand is evidently striving to resuscitate the moribund glamour of two intersecting power-structures that have lost prestige in the Popular Mind for failing to 'wipe out the disease'. Conflated in his canvas, like the earthly and heavenly planes in a relic-laden shrine, are the Medical Establishment militant here on earth and the British Monarchy entrusted by heaven with the defence of the faith.

'Votive Offering' boggles the mind with its advanced aesthetic celebration of the culturally retrograde. Its political design could not be more arcanely patriarchal: the principle of white male unity and supremacy (St George) towers over the divided and dependent female self (Sunnye and Diana) through whom the power of Christ is mediated to the privileged Medical Establishment (Sunnye's father in the guise of a doctor) and thence to the marginalized gay community (the chorus of eroticized PWAs) and finally to the inferiorized Third World (St Sebastian as the embodiment of Black Africa). This is the same rigidly stratified universe mentally inhabited by the religious readers of the tabloids. As an icon of that world, 'Votive Offering' is just the heavenly side of the coin offered by the *Weekly World News*; flip it, and we're back in the Hell Hospital at Los Cocos.

THE FOUNTAIN OF BLOOD

Martyrs are made, not born, and their makers tend to revel in the potent symbolism of blood to promote agendas that often have little to do with the lives and aspirations of the venerated dead. In the *Weekly World News* we saw the Nurse from Hell diverting the River of Life from the veins of the Los Cocos victims into Science's endless plastic tubes; in 'Votive Offering' we saw those same tubes hooked up to blood bags on the IV stands in the Shrine of the Royal Touch. Surely for years to come we can expect fountains of blood to flow in the representations of the AIDS martyrium.

There's a gusher, for instance, in the opening pages of June Callwood's *Jim: A Life With AIDS* (1988). As the first full-blown saint's life in the AIDS canon, this painfully allegorical work is the prose counterpart to 'Votive Offering'.[17] Though it was marketed as a biography of PWA Jim Zanuck – 'Canada's longest surviving AIDS patient' – it hardly qualifies as non-fiction, since blood imagery colours its 310 pages with the dark crimson of martyrological fantasy. The name Zanuck, we learn, was invented by Callwood to cloak her celebrity subject's real identity. As for his other surname, St James, he invented it himself for professional reasons during his career as an actor in Toronto. This gaily ironic stage name has made canonization relatively easy for his straight biographers.

The 'Vita Sancti Jacobi' was briefly told before Callwood by Eileen Whitfield in an article for a glossy Toronto magazine. Entitled 'Witness', the article dwelt upon Jim's painful upbringing as a Jehovah's Witness, but it also implicitly proclaimed him a martyr in the original Christian sense, a charismatic witness to the strength of the Spirit facing the frailty of the Flesh.

JAMES MILLER

Whitfield's subtitle spelled out her inspirational theme: 'Jim St James, the Canadian who's survived the longest with AIDS, has made his peace with sex, death, and religion.'[18]

If only that were so! It was June Callwood's mission to present his very worldly 'Life with AIDS' (the grim parody of an other-worldly 'Life with Christ') as an agony without closure, a continuing no-exit martyrdom in which the self-sainted actor finds himself caught between the warring legions of the Flesh and the Spirit and never makes peace with sex, death, religion, or anything else. Flesh and Spirit were ferociously dualized in his mind long before Callwood set the petty bourgeois details of his life against the profoundly violent backdrop of the Conflict of the Soul.[19] Since she never criticizes Jim's crypto-gnostic view of the world, at least not in print, she effectively colluded with him in promoting his primitive eschatology as the key to understanding all AIDS mythologies. In this respect she ironically replaced Jim's own mother, a die-hard Witness who will never write an Anglican-style 'Mother's Story' since she has zealously refused to communicate with her son since his double coming out as a gay PWA.

In her introduction, Callwood says that she expected he would die before the book was finished. (When he finally did die, in the winter of 1990, it was a good two years after his life was wrapped up in her book.) 'Several times that summer when I left him after hours of taping interviews,' she recalls, 'I would flee to Casey House to weep on the first sympathetic shoulder I could find.'[20]

The Mater Dolorosa of Casey House, the Toronto AIDS hospice she founded, Callwood was caught in an ironic bind. As a writer under contract to fashion this actor's life into something universally meaningful, she needed his death to determine her deadline. But the promised end that would have crowned his militant life kept eluding her, as she admits in her introduction. Imagine the frustration of an avid martyrologist stuck with a martyr who simply couldn't die – not even by his own hand. There was only one thing to do: *kill him off symbolically* at the start of the book so that everything following his 'death' in the plotting of the story can be read as a moralized reconstruction of his life as an 'exemplum' of heroic courage in the face of cruel persecution. The symbolic killing had to be sacrificial and voluntary, of course, if her victim was to qualify for a crown, but it also had to have buckets of blood – real blood – if his victory over the Flesh was to satisfy the first condition of martyrdom. Within the first three pages of Chapter 1 she succeeds in constructing an allegorical scene in which Jim fulfils all three conditions of martyrdom without even knowing it.

Marvel we must at Callwood's lead-in to the opening scene, a mini-psychomachia presented in the assessment-file style familiar to readers of pop-psychology manuals. During the day Jim lived the role of a godly celibate, immersing himself in his religion and studying his Bible; at night, however, he would weep in despair, praying God to forgive his homosexuality. Needless to

67

say, these periods of religious fervour would be followed by episodes of 'wanton promiscuity'.[21]

Callwood's diction often betrays an unacknowledged collusion with the Witnesses, whose 'stern religion' (as she calls it) condemns Jim to the tedium of street-corner proselytizing and endless head-knocking monologues with a Supreme Being quite unable to transcend the sexual mores of the 1950s – not to mention the fifth century. 'Stern' hardly begins to describe a religion that would compel a mother (as it compelled Jim's) to denounce her son as he writhed in pain, riddled with cancer, on the 'moral grounds' that as a gay PWA he was beyond the charmed circle of Jehovah's family! Such inflexible bigotry isn't high moral sternness: it's just lowbrow conservative familialism raised to the heights of apocalyptic paranoia.

How could Callwood, a professed advocate for gay PWAs, tolerate the punitive homophobia of this neo-Manichaean sect so blandly in her book? Did she fear Ayatollah-style reprisals from terrorist Witnesses? Or was their fierce moral absolutism somehow *required* by the hagiographical design of her story as a corrective to permissive liberal relativism? Instead of describing the other side of Jim's divided life as an eager affirmation of gay identity or even as a relaxing break from hours of fruitless Bible study, she represents it just as the Witnesses surely would, as a fling 'into wanton promiscuity'. Jim was evidently not born with Callwood's appreciation of the Golden Mean: her exquisite sense of just how many sexual partners it takes before you're disfellowshipped from decent society and cast down into the circle of the sluts.

When AIDS makes itself apparent on Jim's skin – that public screen where the Sins of the Flesh are projected for all to see and condemn – it functions as an answer to his Old Testament fist-shaking. Two hard lumps appear on his head like the boils of Job or the mark of Cain. When he consults a skin specialist about their removal, he is told to call back in a month, but Jim can't wait that long. His career as an actor is just taking off; within a year he will be playing Don Quixote in an amateur production of *Man of La Mancha*, for which he will receive a Theatre Ontario award – along with his AIDS diagnosis. So he reveals much later in his taped confessions. But at the time of his first lumps he knew nothing of God's Plan.

Callwood's plan, however, is plain enough at this early point in her tale. She is already setting up a symbolic antithesis between the two cultural institutions dominating Jim's Life: the other-worldly Church and the ultra-worldly Theatre, just as the Late Antique martyrologists pitted the showbiz culture of Old Rome against the redemptive cult of the New Jerusalem. Any normal worldling, worried about his looks for professional reasons, would have waited a month or two for a qualified surgeon and a hygienic operating room. But not Jim. As a saint caught in the unhygienic embrace of the Theatre, he cannot wait to purge himself of unclean thoughts and unclean

tissue. That same day, without benefit of anaesthesia, he boldly attempts an auto-lumpectomy in his bathroom.

Fortitude (rather than intelligence) always was the virtue of martyrs, and Jim displays it here in abundance. His symbolic flaying, a crude rite of fleshly mortification, serves as his initiation into the agony of AIDS treatments, and he may be forgiven some initial astonishment at its impact on his circulatory system: 'His face was covered in blood, blood dripping from his chin, blood soaking the bathroom mat.' Blood on the mat? There's a detail to distress suburban readers who spend so much of their lives maintaining spic-and-span bathrooms, but its goriness is necessary here to shock just such people into a Late Antique awareness of the blood-drenched tides of mortality. Just think how absorbent those mats are: clearly this is no mere flesh wound but a deep gash into the Collective Unconscious (also known as the Popular Mind), where blood is simultaneously informed with immanent divinity and demonic virulence.

Jim is transfixed by his wound, his red badge of courage, perhaps because it is a sign of his emergent identity as an AIDS martyr. Unflinchingly, as if fingering the stigmata, he touches the incision. Eventually an ice pack staunches the flow of blood – but not for long. As if driven by the insatiably gory conventions of martyr discourse itself, Jim is soon seeking out another bathroom for another bloodbath. A few days later, at his lover Paul's apartment, he discovers that the cyst has returned, 'protruding from his scalp like a balloon'.[22]

Don't touch it for God's sake, the queasy reader is inclined to shout; but for the sake of Jehovah God, Jim must detonate the viral bomb. As a martyr in the making he has no more desire to stop the horrible purgation of his sins than does a hero in a horror film (so dictated by literary conventions is his fictional will) to enter the creepy passageway into the vampire's crypt. Martyrs and vampires are peculiarly alike in their compulsive bloodlust. Both achieve immortality through quasi-erotic effusions of bodily fluid. Both perversely triumph over death.

Should Callwood's readers wonder whether Jim will turn out to be a martyr or a vampire in Chapter 1, the dénouement of the cyst scene surely resolves any doubt about our hero's saintly status. Jim looks at the cyst in the mirror and touches it gently, whereupon it explodes 'in a fountain of blood'. Fully clothed, he turns on the shower to wash it away. Ordinarily, when someone's bubble bursts, it means an end to his worldly ambitions. But not here: this is Jim's big break. In the years of AIDS treatments to come he will act out the self-deluded yet oddly heroic part of the martyr-knight, the Don Quixote of Sunnybrook Hospital. Callwood dreams the impossible dream with him, and makes him a hero in her own apocalyptic drama of dissolution and resurrection. Immanent divinity is an offer no Jehovah's Witness can refuse, and in the tropological subtext of this crucial opening scene our hero

implicitly accepts it by confronting the frailty of his Flesh in the mirror of Worldly Vanity.

Why did Callwood describe this second effusion as 'a fountain of blood'? Why not a spurt, or simply a lot of blood? I suspect that she was echoing (no doubt unconsciously) the following sanguinary lines from a favourite anthem of the old-time-religion set –

> There is a fountain filled with blood,
> Drawn from Emmanuel's veins;
> And sinners, plunged beneath that flood,
> Lose all their guilty stains.[23]

By flooding his lover's bathroom with the currents of his agonized heart, and then plunging beneath the shower to wipe away the guilty stains of his gayness, Jim figuratively identifies himself with the Pure at Heart and thus perfects his quixotic role as a chivalric imitator of Christ.

People rarely bleed fountains or bathe in them unless they happen to be bona fide Grail Knights or mental inhabitants of the Holy Grail universe (as Don Quixote was), forever in quest of the ultimate victory for a Soldier of Christ – the victory over Death. The knights and martyrs in the Ghent Altarpiece, for instance, triumph over Death *en masse* by marching towards the garden of the Fountain of Life where the Lamb of God bleeds into a chalice.[24] Like these winners in the race for immortality, Callwood's bleeding knight errant was quaintly and preposterously prepared 'to march into hell for a heavenly cause' (namely the War on AIDS) by becoming his own healing saint, an apotheosized presence enshrined in the Casey House martyrium.[25] Far from making the gay PWA a socially accessible human being, Callwood transforms him into a remote star in her apocalyptic firmament.

Jim's march towards immanent divinity takes him across a moralized landscape that Callwood signposts for all who follow her steps as pilgrims to the shrine of St James. Paradise is the lost homestead of his Southern Ontario boyhood. Purgatory is the Toronto hospital system. As for Hell, it's as easy to spot on Callwood's mental map as Los Cocos was on the map in the *Weekly World News*. Jim locates it for us in the Gay Underworld of New York, which 'presented him with sexual depravity beyond anything he had ever known, even in Toronto's roughest S & M community'. On the brighter side, Hell offered him 'such imaginative and luxurious discos as the Saint, with its planetarium ceiling of stars and a magnificent mirror bar crowned with huge flower arrangements'.[26]

What possible harm can come to Jim at an upscale disco like the Saint? It sounds like the perfect venue for him; with its starry ceiling it even looks like Heaven. But beware: all Hell breaks loose in the Disco of the Damned with the coming of the viral anti-Christ. With an almost Spenserian sensitivity to the moral dangers of glitz, Callwood observes that Jim 'loved the opulence

and *lowered* himself into it joyfully' (emphasis mine): his Fall from the heights of respectable middle-class taste, epitomized by the Edenic homestead in Ontario, into the perilous embrace of 'opulence', teaches us all to avoid sex anywhere near magnificent mirror bars and huge flower arrangements.[27]

If the trumpet shall sound and the dead shall be raised, we may be sure that Jim St James will be raised incorruptible – since Callwood has virtually washed away all spot of fleshly corruption from his sacred memory. 'Although I am sleeping in front of you now,' the Witness promises in his taped will, 'I will come back to you through the promise of the resurrection that the God of the Bible made.'[28] On this eerie note, which sounds like an official ecclesiastical transcript of the dead saint's voice, mysteriously emanating from his imaginary tomb in the Casey House martyrium, the Saint's Life draws to its messianic close.

Incorruptible martyrs cannot exist apart from corruptible ideologies, however, even after they've been washed in the Blood of the Lamb. They must always be martyrs *to* something – often not to their own causes but to those of the saintmakers. Since Callwood could advocate neither the punitive fundamentalism of the Jehovah's Witnesses nor the radical erotics of Gay Liberation – the two opposing religions he himself tried to live – she takes the middle course and ironically entombs him amid the gay 'carnage' on the viral battlefield as a witness to her own philanthropic liberalism.

There's no known cure for Acquired Immanent Divinity Syndrome, since those who spread it through casual contact with the complex theology of beatification think they're immune to supernatural solicitings. But criticism of its insidious impact on PWAs who don't want the burden of sainthood may act, perhaps, as a socially effective vaccine.

The chief advantage of martyr discourse for AIDS commentators is that it offers everyone a victorious way out of the victim debate. Radical activists, retrograde artists, reactionary administrators, even reasonable Anglicans have recruited the AIDS dead as martyrs to this or that cause in order to undo their deaths, to keep their spirit 'alive' or their image 'fresh' in the Popular Mind. But a way out of something is always a way into something else – unless you're moving in circles. As with motion, so with argument: if martyr discourse is truly an exit from Shilts's mass market and Watney's mass grave, then it must also be an entry into some region of ironic or paradoxical agreement beyond the darkling plain where reactionaries count their blessings and radicals count their dead.

The chief disadvantage of martyr discourse for AIDS commentators who want to keep hopes up during the crisis without provoking a revival of old-time religion is that it *is* old-time religion. By 'old' I mean really old – not just plague-ravaged medieval but demon-crazy Late Antique. It is the Christian equivalent of the old-time Islamic religion revived with ferocious energy by the Ayatollah Khomeini, who was not one to take martyr discourse lightly.

He literally built it into the design of a Tehran military cemetery by constructing a fountain of blood ('a coloured-water memorial') to commemorate and perpetuate the glorious sacrifice of Iranian youths to the Shi'ite cause in his holy war against Iraq.[29]

Whether the martyrologists of the AIDS crisis realize it or not, they are forcing PWAs to march across a violently apocalyptic terrain, dragging a holy mountain of eschatological baggage. We would do well, then, before martyr discourse becomes the dominant mode of constructing the AIDS narrative, to consider where it might take us and what it might do to the people living with AIDS who want to do so in peace, yet find themselves having to fight the Good Fight to the death in arenas not of their own making.

NOTES

[1]On the 'medical gaze', see Michel Foucault, *The Birth of the Clinic: An Archeology of Medical Perception*, trans A.M. Sheridan (New York: Random House, 1975), pp. 107-23.

[2]For instance, conservative columnist William F. Buckley Jr., who has recommended that all people who test positive for HIV antibodies be tattooed for convenient identification. See his notorious article 'Identify All the Carriers', *New York Times*, 27 May 1986. For a refutation of Buckley's 'tortured argument', see Allan M. Brandt, *No Magic Bullet: A Social History of Venereal Disease in the United States Since 1880* (Oxford and New York: Oxford University Press, 1987), p. 196.

[3]"Founding Statement of People with AIDS/ARC (The Denver Principles)', cited in *AIDS: Cultural Analysis/Cultural Activism*, ed. Douglas Crimp, *October* 43 (Winter 1987): 148.

[4]Randy Shilts, *And the Band Played On: Politics, People, and the AIDS Epidemic* (New York: St Martin's Press, 1987), p. 315. On Shilts's novelistic strategies see James Miller, 'AIDS in the Novel: Getting It Straight', in *Break the Fatal Silence: Artists and Critics in the AIDS Crisis*, ed. James Miller (Toronto: University of Toronto Press, forthcoming).

[5]Michael Callen recommends vigorous scepticism as an effective therapy for PWAs throughout his radically upbeat manual *Surviving and Thriving with AIDS* (cited in Crimp, p. 166): 'If I believed everything I was told, if I believed that tiresome boilerplate that AIDS is "100 percent fatal", then I'd probably be dead by now. . . . If I didn't arm myself with information, with diverse views, I would be unable to defend myself from the madness and gibberish that daily assault those of us who have acquired immune deficiency syndrome.'

[6]Shilts, p. 425.

[7]Simon Watney, *Policing Desire: Pornography, AIDS and the Media* (Minneapolis: University of Minnesota Press, 1987), p. 147.

[8]Ibid., p. 148.

[9]The analogy between AIDS and the Holocaust was articulated and popularized by Larry Kramer in his political drama *The Normal Heart* (New York: New American

Library, 1985). 'Did you ever consider it could get so bad they'll quarantine us or put us in camps?' cries Kramer's outraged gay activist hero Ned Weeks (II.13, p. 113): 'It's happened before. It's all happened before. History is worth shit. I swear to God I now understand. . . . Is this how so many people just walked into gas chambers?'

[10]The source for most modern Catholic discussions of the conditions for martyrdom is Thomas Aquinas's 'Of Martyrdom', *Summa Theologica* Part II, question cxxiv, articles 1-5. For a translation of this passage see *The "Summa Theologica" of St Thomas Aquinas*, vol. 12 (London: Burns Oates and Washbourne, 1922, 1935), pp. 215-26.

[11]'Living with AIDS, and Death: What am I?' by 'David', *The Anglican Magazine* (October 1987): 5-6. Despite his radical allegiance to the Gay Movement, David still perceives his plight in fundamentally bleak Old Testament terms. 'My mother didn't want me to write the article, perhaps for my sake as well as hers,' he confesses: 'I don't think it is easy to lose your *firstborn* child . . .' (my emphasis). Since he evidently perceives himself as a Passover sacrifice, it's no wonder that he conceives AIDS as a hideously ironic plague perpetrated on gays by the wrathful God of Moses. This conception of the epidemic both angers and consoles him. One moment he rejects the victim role on gay political grounds. The next he embraces it – provided that it is interpreted religiously in relation to sacrificial honour and divine justice. His chief regret: 'I really didn't get enough time to experience "gay liberation" before I was a victim of "gay plague".'

[12]'A Mother's Story', ed. John Bird, *The Anglican Magazine* (October 1987): 8.

[13]In the Sistine 'Last Judgement', St Bartholomew holds up his flayed skin like Veronica's veil, bearing, it is thought, an image of Michelangelo's face to suggest the painter's heroic self-martyrdom in the agony of artistic creation.

[14]In a conversation with Horsley in the spring of 1989, I learned that he has only recently come to regard his triptych as an 'AIDS painting'. His original intention in 1987 (when he conceived and completed its design) was to produce a work celebrating Gay Liberation as a counter–discourse to repressive Christian teachings on the body as the locus of sinful pleasures, sadistic torments, and demonic invasions. It was not until the summer of 1988 that he began to regard the work as peculiarly 'relevant to the epidemic' after learning that the two men portrayed in the outer panels had both received positive results on an HIV-antibody test.

[15]For a photograph of Sunnye as an AIDS victim proving that 'now no one is safe', see the cover of *Life* (July 1985).

[16]On the symbolic significance of the location and structure of the martyrium in Late Antiquity and the Middle Ages, see Peter Brown, *The Cult of the Saints* (Chicago: University of Chicago Press, 1981), pp. 8-9, 21, 86-91.

[17]Callwood's chief rival in the PWA biography line is Paul Monette, whose memoir of Roger Horwitz's life with AIDS – *Borrowed Time* (San Diego and New York: Harcourt Brace Jovanovich, 1988) – carefully avoids martyr discourse. Alienated as a gay man from mainstream American Christianity, Monette returns to the nineteenth-century discourse of classical tragedy in his efforts to immortalize his beloved: e.g., 'Perhaps the world is always full of portents, as the oracle

maintained it was, in every flight of birds that passes. The only thing we could do to hold the fates at bay was to keep our own world full to the brim . . .' (p. 24).

[18] Eileen Whitfield, 'Witness', *Saturday Night* (January 1988): 36-42.

[19] The Greek term 'psychomachia' literally means 'soul-war': i.e., a conflict in the soul between fleshly desires and spiritual aspirations. The late Latin poet Prudentius (c. 400 AD) used the term as the title for a long allegorical poem in which personified Virtues and Vices struggle for possession of the human soul. For a translation of the *Psychomachia*, see *Prudentius*, vol. 1, ed. H.J. Thomson (London: William Heinemann, 1949), pp. 274-343.

[20] June Callwood, *Jim: A Life with AIDS* (Toronto: Lester and Orpen Dennys, 1988), p. 3.

[21] Ibid., p. 6.

[22] Ibid., p. 7.

[23] Lyric (based on Zechariah 13:1) by William Cowper, *The Methodist Hymnal* (Nashville: The Methodist Publishing House, 1964, 1966), no. 421.

[24] On the symbolic connection between the Fountain of Life and the Blood of the Lamb, see Lotte Brand Philip, *The Ghent Altarpiece and the Art of Jan van Eyck* (Princeton: Princeton University Press, 1971), pp. 66-70.

[25] 'The Impossible Dream', line 12, from *Man of La Mancha* (words by Joe Darrion, music by Mitch Leigh: Andrew Scott Inc, Helena Music Co, 1965). By reprinting the entire text of this song at a critical moment in her narrative – just when Jim receives his Theatre Ontario award and his AIDS diagnosis (*Jim: A Life with AIDS*, pp. 136-7) – Callwood turns it into a grotesquely ironic gloss on her hero's far from romantic life. Unhappily Jim finds his Dulcinea in a rich but reckless Jehovah's Witness virgin named Iris Hrabovsky, whom he marries briefly in the mid-1970s. When heterosexual bliss proves to be an impossible dream for him, he simply switches roles from dutiful husband to gay Prodigal Son and heads for the wicked discos of New York.

[26] Callwood, *Jim: A Life with AIDS*, pp. 117-19.

[27] Ibid., p. 119. So parable-like is Jim's life with AIDS that even in his life before AIDS he could hardly enter a store without transforming it into an allegorical locus of demonic depravity and sexual temptation. I shudder to think what the managers of Eaton's, Toronto's most respectable WASP department store, thought when they read Callwood's account of Jim's erotic experiences in the display department of their old College Street building, where his lust amid the mannikins compelled him now and then to masturbate (fortunately not in the display windows). Colluding with his own direly moralistic interpretation of this act, Callwood remarks that when he was finished masturbating he felt devastated: 'What he had done was wrong, demonic, bad, evil' (p. 78).

[28] Ibid., p. 310. At Jim's memorial service, Callwood read excerpts from the transcript of his taped will.

[29] For a photograph of this memorial, see *Time* (17 Nov. 1986): 30.

SEXUAL ETHICS AND AIDS:
A LIBERAL VIEW

MICHAEL YEO

AIDS AND SEXUAL MORALIZING

AIDS has been socially constructed according to moral categories in a way that few other illness have ever been. It has been widely regarded as a sign of immorality and even a punishment for moral transgression. People with AIDS have been stigmatized, scorned, and shunned as 'moral lepers'.

The dynamics of this process are easy enough to understand. Sex has always been a leading preoccupation of moralists, and when AIDS first appeared in the early 1980s it quickly became a target for moralizing because of its association with sex. Homosexuality, promiscuity, prostitution, and extra-marital sex, foremost among the 'cardinal sins' of the flesh, happen also to have become associated with AIDS.[1] The moralizing directed against these 'moral transgressions' came to be directed as well against AIDS: guilt by association.

From the start, I want to dissociate my analysis of AIDS and sexual ethics from the sexual moralizing that has been so pervasive in relation to AIDS.[2] In the first place, I am deeply suspicious about the way the 'cardinal sins' identified above have come to be designated as such. In matters of sexuality, right is typically distinguished from wrong with reference to less overtly normative distinctions, such as those between natural v. unnatural, normal v. perverted, sex with love v. without love, open to procreation v. not open to procreation, and so on. When pressed to justify moral claims about sex, people often respond by saying things to the effect that such and such a sexual practice is wrong *because* it is unnatural, or perverted, or occurs without love, or is not open to procreation. This 'because' raises more questions than it answers.

In the second place, to the extent that it is fruitful to analyse sexual ethics along these lines, AIDS adds nothing to the argument. The claim, popular with some moralists, that AIDS 'proves' that homosexuality is morally wrong requires (at the very least) the premise that nature is somehow constituted in such a way as to punish so-called immoral behaviour. Even if sense could be made of this claim, one would be faced with the troubling anomaly that at least some of the people thus 'punished' – haemophiliacs and infants – are not by the moralist's standards 'guilty'.

Finally, and most importantly, the moralizing line of thinking does nothing to illuminate the specific sorts of issues that AIDS raises in sexual ethics. Worse still, it tends to be applied in ways that unjustly victimize and villainize people living with AIDS or under its shadow.

AIDS, SEX, AND INFORMED CONSENT

The approach I shall take, by contrast, could be termed 'liberal'[3] insofar as it remains neutral with respect to the categories of sexual moralizing and instead relies on the idea of consent as a touchstone for distinguishing right from wrong in sexual matters. The standard here could be stated as follows:

> The morality of a given sexual activity is to be judged in accordance with whether those involved have freely consented to participate.

Sexual activity that takes place without consent is wrong for that reason. It may also be wrong for other sorts of reasons, but that is something about which a liberal approach remains neutral. In analysing the morality of a given sexual activity or involvement according to this standard, questions as to whether the activity is 'natural' or 'normal', or 'occurs in the context of a loving relationship', and so on, are not relevant, or are relevant only insofar as they might have some bearing on whether those involved have consented to be so.

I do not propose to offer any justification for this standard, which would be quite beyond the scope of this paper and would take us some distance from the topic of AIDS. For my limited purposes, it should be enough to explain why I think it is an especially appropriate starting point for analysing sexual ethics and AIDS. In the first place, whether one approves of the standard or not, it comes closer than any other I can think of to reflecting the sexual ethic that is in practice most pervasive in our society, and certainly among those who are most sexually active and therefore most at risk of contracting HIV infection through sexual transmission.[4] Moreover, I think that even people with less 'permissive' standards will accept this as being at least a minimal standard. Second, this standard, it will be shown, is of some help in analysing the kinds of issues that AIDS raises in relation to sexual ethics, and in particular matters having to do with self-disclosure and truth-telling.

In some ways this is a simple standard, but the concept of consent is by no means simple. I will explicate this concept with reference to the literature in bioethics, where it has undergone considerable scrutiny. The analogy between sexual and biomedical relationships might seem at first glance absurd (and at some level it is), but will appear less so if one considers how intimately one's body may come to be known in each case, and that in a time of AIDS the risk of harm arising out of sexual encounters may be comparable to that in many medical encounters.

Ethicists analyse consent into two aspects, one pertaining to the voluntariness of the consent and the other to the knowledge informing it: hence the phrase 'informed consent'.[5] The requirement of voluntariness has no special bearing on AIDS *per se*. Everyone will agree that it is wrong to involve someone in sex involuntarily or coercively. To be sure, there are grey areas – for example, whether someone 'driven' into a sexual encounter by passion or lust is truly acting voluntarily – but AIDS introduces no new shades here. The requirement that consent be properly informed, however, does have a direct bearing on ethical issues arising in connection with AIDS, to which I now turn.

Many ethical issues surrounding AIDS have to do with the disclosure of information about whether person X has AIDS or is HIV-positive,[6] or even whether he or she is a member of some class of people statistically more susceptible to HIV-infection. Does X have a duty to convey such information to anyone? If so, to whom and for what reasons? Does anyone have a right to expect or demand this information from X, or from others who might be privy to it? Analysis of such questions requires consideration of certain empirical factors, the most important of these being the extent to which X puts others at risk. If I am not being put at risk in virtue of my involvement with X (for example, X is selling me a car), there is no obvious reason why I ought to know any AIDS-related information about X, or why X ought to tell me.

The matter appears in a different light in situations where X does put someone at risk. Fortunately, HIV is not easily transmitted from one person to another, and the kinds of activities or involvements by which someone is put at risk are few in number and easily identifiable. Sexual activity is foremost among these. Looking at sexual ethics from the standpoint of informed consent, it is reasonable to expect that knowledge of risk and of the extent to which someone may be putting me at risk might have some bearing on my consent to a given sexual involvement.

Generally speaking, risk of getting HIV infection varies according to two factors: what you are doing, and who you are doing it with. With respect to the former, the risk classification system proposed in the Canadian AIDS Society's *Safer Sex Guidelines*, although by no means uncontroversial, should suffice for my purposes.[7] This guide groups sexual activities under three main risk headings: 'no possibility of HIV transmission', 'minimal to low possibility', and 'very high possibility'. This classification is based on the assumption that the person with whom you are having sex is actually HIV-infectious. If your sexual partner is not infectious, the risk to you is zero, regardless of the sexual activity. Of course, it may be practically impossible to know this for certain, and this is why the *Guidelines* advise us to assume the worst for the purpose of regulating our behaviour, and thus to act as if others were HIV-infectious (except under very specific conditions to be discussed later).

Risk also varies depending on whom one is having sex with, however, or, more precisely, depending on the probability of his or her being infectious. The greater this probability, the more risky will be any sexual involvement open to HIV transmission. A high-risk sexual activity – unprotected inter-course, for example – will be all the more risky if it involves someone with a high probability of being infectious – an intravenous drug-user living in Vancouver who habitually shares needles, let us say.

The concept of 'risk groups', however, is controversial. As *Guidelines* points out, it is frequently used to stigmatize people already marginalized in our society.[8] This is not a sufficient reason to abandon use of the concept altogether, but it does place an onus on those who would use it to do so responsibly and to be clear about how and why it is being applied. In connection with sexual ethics, two applications might come into play. First, the concept is relevant for the purpose of sorting out duties to others in the context of sexual relations. A good case can be made that people who know themselves to be in a high-risk group – at the limit, people who know for a fact that they are HIV-positive – have special duties by way of not harming others: e.g., to practise safer sex. One might respond that, with few excep-tions, everyone should be practising safer sex anyway, but even so there is a moral difference between practising safer sex for reasons of self-protection and doing so for reasons of protecting others. Only the second is what we would normally consider a duty, and it is a duty that bears on some people in our society more than on others.

Second, and much more problematically, the concept of risk groups might figure in some kind of screening strategy used by individuals seeking to protect themselves from infection. That is, someone might rely on AIDS-related information about a prospective partner for purposes of deciding what kinds of sexual activity, if any, to engage in with that person. This strategy, as *Guidelines* convincingly argues, may be tragically imprudent.[9] As a matter of fact, the signs by which to assess the probability of membership in a high-risk group are unreliable. Moreover, the inference that a prospective partner is 'safe' because he or she does not (or so one might think) fall into any so-called high-risk group is unwarranted, since HIV is by no means restricted to people in high-risk groups. It is for these sorts of reasons that *Guidelines* advises that the best way of protecting oneself (and others) is to practise safer sex. These arguments notwithstanding, however, there is some value in knowing AIDS-related information about sexual partners, and *Guidelines* explicitly acknowledges this in the context of so-called monogamous relationships. For the time being, I will take the value of such information as given, and later will argue the case in the context of defending the approach advocated here against objections.

Given this background, let us turn to some specific issues that AIDS raises in connection with sexual ethics. These issues have to do mainly with information-sharing and truth-telling. What AIDS-related information about myself am I obliged to disclose to a sexual partner? What information does that person have a right to expect from me?

Analysed in terms of the model of informed consent, the issue centres around what in biomedical contexts is called the 'standard of disclosure' for consent.[10] This standard gives guidance for determining what kind of information, and how much of it, is necessary in order for a given consent to be truly an *informed* consent. The standard of disclosure I propose as a general rule with respect to consent in matters sexual is as follows:

> People are obliged to disclose to sexual partners any such AIDS-related information about themselves as would be germane to the decision of a reasonable person to be sexually involved with them.

Using this standard, the burden of analysis is shifted onto the notion of 'reasonable person'. This is a controversial notion, but we can make some relatively uncontroversial assumptions about what would be germane to the consent of a reasonable person in such matters.[11] Certainly consideration of risk would have a bearing on a reasonable person's consent to sexual involvement, and the greater the risk the greater the bearing it would have on the consent. Risk in turn is a function both of sexual activity – no risk, minimal to low risk, high risk – and of the probability of one's partner being infectious. The reasonable person considering sexual activity with me would want to know if I was HIV-positive by way of making an informed choice about sexual involvement with me, even assuming that the reasonable person would also be practising safer sex (safer sex is not entirely risk-free).[12] Moreover, I think my obligation to disclose this would be the more imperative the riskier the sexual activity to take place.

The reasonable person standard becomes more problematic as we move from the case where someone knows he or she is HIV-infectious to the case where the individual knows only that there is a high probability of this. Statistically speaking, for example, if I am a male who has a history of frequent unsafe sexual encounters with people in the gay community in Toronto (perhaps I have since learned that some of these same people now have AIDS), the probability that I am infectious is considerably higher than the statistical average. Am I obliged to disclose to prospective sexual partners my membership in a so-called 'high-risk group'?

This question is debatable, and all the more so the lower the probability of my being infectious and the lower the risk of the sexual activity to take place. Suppose, for example, that I have a history of unsafe behaviour – needle-sharing or unprotected sex – in a community in which the incidence of HIV infection is very high, and have recently entered into an as yet non-sexual relationship with a woman unaware of this. Am I obliged to disclose such AIDS-related information before engaging her in sexual activity that would put her at risk?[13]

This example highlights the relevance of contextual factors to informed consent. Insofar as we know something about the determinate context in light of which *this particular person* might give or fail to give consent, additional 'subjective' or context-specific considerations beyond the reasonable person standard must be brought into play in the analysis. What would be germane to the consent of *this particular person in this particular set of circumstances*? For example, a good case can be made that, if I know she is under the mistaken assumption I am 'safe', I am obliged to inform her otherwise. Granted, she may be naïve or foolish to make such an assumption, but even so her consent to sexual activity with me would be given in light of this understanding. To the extent that this is a misunderstanding, her consent would be uninformed, and I would be negligent if I failed to disclose AIDS-related information about myself that would correct her misunderstanding. Moreover, I would be all the more culpable the more deliberately I exploited or promoted such misunderstanding, and the more risky the sexual activity that might ensue. The case for disclosure is even more compelling if my partner actively seeks AIDS-related information from me in order to determine the probability of risk of involvement with me. In this event, failure to disclose would amount to lying in one form or another, and consent obtained by means of deception is clearly invalid.

The idea of informed consent does not furnish a mechanical formula for resolving all truth-telling issues that might arise in connection with sex and AIDS. It has to be *interpreted* with reference to the particulars of the case at hand, taking into consideration the degree of risk and the nature of the understanding in light of which consent to sexual activity might take place. It does, however, provide a fruitful framework within which to analyse the issues. In some cases, this analysis will be fairly straightforward, and the obligation regarding disclosure more or less uncontroversial. In others, there will be more room for interpretation and debate about what amount of disclosure, ethically speaking, is required. A certain amount of imprecision is inherent in ethical analysis in matters of conduct. As Aristotle says, 'it is the mark of an educated mind to expect that amount of exactness in each kind which the nature of the particular subject admits.'[14]

In any event, I have said enough to convey the general style of analysis along these lines. It remains to consider some fundamental objections to this approach, since if the approach is fundamentally flawed, arguments about how it ought to be applied in a given case are, in the worst sense of the word, academic.

THREE OBJECTIONS TO THE INFORMED-CONSENT APPROACH

The first objection to be considered concerns the requirement of voluntariness implicit in the idea of informed consent. Sexual interactions, it might be argued, are notoriously motivated by passion, and seldom follow upon deliberate prior thought. This being so, is it really appropriate to analyse sexual interactions in terms of consent, let alone *informed* consent? The problem here has a parallel in the medical arena, from which the doctrine of informed consent is derived. Not infrequently, treatment decisions must be made very quickly, under conditions of extreme stress and emotion, and with regard to medical matters about which patients may know very little. The quality of the consent may be compromised, but even so we apply the idea of informed consent to such situations. To be sure, in extreme cases we deem the decision-maker 'incompetent' to decide, but normally this is done because of what is thought to be some cognitive impairment. The mere presence of strong emotions or passions is not sufficient to warrant pronouncing someone incompetent.

In any event, I would concede that the passionate moment is not the best time during which to engage in rational discussion about sex, but would emphasize that it is also not the only time during which such discussion might take place. The threat of AIDS (one might argue along similar lines about the 'threat of pregnancy') is serious enough to cause us to pause and think about how we ought best to comport ourselves in these matters *before* we find ourselves caught in the throes of the passionate moment. The passionate moment may indeed compromise rational thinking and voluntariness, but this is all the more reason why such thinking should take place prior to the passionate moment, and why one should make some decisions in advance.

The voluntariness of sexual activity may also be compromised by relations of power. Participants in sexual activity are not always operating on a level playing field (the same could be said of health-care professionals and patients). As Canadian AIDS-educator Kate Hankins has pointed out, 'the majority of women at higher risk for HIV acquisition don't have the power within sexual relationships to negotiate a change in the rules.'[15] This is sadly true, but the fact that the voluntariness of sex is often compromised by relations of power does not militate against applying the standard of informed consent to sexual relationships. Indeed, it is because we do so that we take involuntary or coercive sex to be wrong.

Moreover, if thinking about sexual relationships in terms of informed consent were to become more prevalent in our society, it could play a role in empowering those caught up in less than fully autonomous sexual relationships. Informed consent requires discussion, and applied to sexual relationships would mean that people would do a lot more talking about matters bearing on their sexuality and the risks involved. In relationships marked by inequality, it might be appropriate to think of such talk as a kind of negotiation. The idea of people's negotiating sexual relationships – whether to use condoms, for example – as opposed to having the rules of the game unilaterally laid down by the more powerful should be attractive to those who are disempowered.

Such negotiation or discussion, however, is hardly the norm in our society, and there are powerful obstacles standing against it. A major obstacle is the fact that what one might talk about by way of ensuring informed consent is 'taboo',[16] and this no doubt reinforces inequality in sexual relationships. It is noteworthy that the desire to talk about sexual relationships, and specifically to talk about AIDS, appears to be to some degree gender-specific. In a study of AIDS-talk among college students, Sheryl Perlmutter and Paula Michal-Johnson report:

> there are clear differences in the ways men and women approach the issue of AIDS in relationships. Proportionately more of the women in our sample reported talking about AIDS in their relationships. Women seem to want more talk and are likely to take the responsibility for talking about AIDS, particularly as it pertains to their partner's relationship history. Men, on the other hand, are more likely to trust their own observations when assessing potential risks.[17]

Promoting the idea of informed consent in sexual relationships, and therewith promoting increased discussion about AIDS, would strengthen the hand of those typically disempowered in sexual relationships and could help to level the playing field.

A second objection to employing the standard of informed consent in connection with sexual ethics and AIDS concerns the weight that should be given to knowing AIDS-related information about sexual partners. If, as most educators seem to agree, it is advisable to presume for practical purposes that any prospective partner may be infectious, what difference would knowing

AIDS-related information about them make? Why is it important that consent be well-informed?

In the first place, as the authors of the *Safer Sex Guidelines* acknowledge, there is at least one major exception to the general rule that one should always practise safer sex under the presumption that one's partner may be infectious, and that is in monogamous relationships wherein the partners are in fact free of HIV infection.[18] Under such conditions (and it must be emphasized how difficult it is to know with any degree of certainty that such conditions really do obtain) there is no risk of HIV infection, and hence no need or obligation to practise safer sex.

This exception is important in that monogamy, at least in word if not in deed, is highly valued in our society, and is likely to become even more valued in light of the threat of AIDS. In a relationship mistakenly believed by one of the partners to be monogamous and HIV infection-free, there is a special duty to disclose such information as might correct the misunderstanding. In this regard, imagine a couple planning to have a child (and thus unable to avoid sexual activity deemed high-risk according to *Guidelines*). In such situations at least (and especially), AIDS-related information about one's partner would have an obvious bearing on one's choices.

Second, even where safer sex is possible and prudent, screening sexual partners on the basis of their risk status is still a reasonable way to *further* minimize risk. Safer sex, after all, is not 100 per cent safe given the possibility of such contingencies as condom failure or misuse.[19] This risk is admittedly small (in terms of *Guidelines*, sexual intercourse with a condom is classified as 'low-risk'), but even so it would not be unreasonable to decline to take this risk with someone who is or is quite probably HIV-infectious, or perhaps to avoid doing certain things that one might otherwise risk doing.

Finally, and most controversially, one might screen prospective partners *instead* of practising safer sex, or in order to decide when and with whom to practise safer sex. This is completely contrary to the risk-minimization approach advocated in *Guidelines*, and there are several good arguments against it. Even so, however, it is at least an arguable strategy (and some approaches along these lines are no doubt more effective than others), although generally not one I would advocate.[20] Moreover, the fact is that at the present time the majority of people in our society do not as yet practise safer sex and so are especially vulnerable to HIV infection.[21] They may be foolish or imprudent not to do so, but they do not for that reason forfeit their entitlement to moral consideration. Risk-minimization strategies in common use that rely on AIDS-related information about prospective partners are undermined by concealment or deceit, and the quality of the consent of those deceived is seriously compromised.

This last point leads to a third fundamental criticism of approaching sexual ethics and AIDS along the lines of informed consent. It takes two to tango, one might argue, and responsibility for protection ultimately resides with each individual. If people fail to protect themselves – fail to practise safer sex, for example – then it is their 'fault' if they contract HIV from me, even if at the extreme I have knowingly concealed from them that I am infectious. *Caveat emptor!* – 'Buyer beware!' – could be the motto of this approach.   This is an especially serious objection to my argument insofar as it is itself based on liberal grounds. Liberalism, after all, is built on respecting people's freedom to run (and even ruin) their own lives so long as or to the point where their exercise of freedom does not harm others. This also means that others may be excused for exposing me to harm (e.g., selling me a package of cigarettes) if I voluntarily allow myself to be thus exposed.

The approach articulated here is quite consistent with these liberal principles. My rationale for promoting informed consent in connection with sexual ethics, it must be emphasized, is not to prevent people from exposing themselves to harm (although that might be an indirect benefit) but to respect freedom. I accept that there is some onus on 'buyers' to protect themselves in what may be a deadly marketplace, and accept moreover that we ought to respect people's right to expose themselves to risks. However, what I have said about informed consent, far from being incompatible with such freedom and responsibility, is in fact promotive of it. Three points need to be made here.

First of all, as has already been said, screening prospective partners based on information-gathering is a protective strategy. Good arguments could be advanced that it would be more prudent in addition to practise safer sex, but in at least some cases this would be inappropriate (in cases where one plans to have children and therefore cannot avoid what *Guidelines* calls 'high-risk activity', i.e., unprotected vaginal intercourse).

Second, if it can be argued that it is not prudent to screen without also practising safer sex, it can also be argued that it is not prudent to practise safer sex without also screening. Even prudent consumers who avail themselves of the best precautions commercially available assume some risk in engaging in low-risk sexual activity – sexual intercourse with a condom, for example – and, statistically speaking, the risk is greater the greater the probability that one's sexual partner is HIV-infectious. If this probability is high, the consumer is entitled to know this. At the very least, the consumer should not be lied to.

Finally, at this point in time, and no doubt for some time into the future, consumers have not been properly educated about how to protect themselves from AIDS. It is therefore unreasonable to establish safer sex practices as the standard of care to which people should be expected to conform, however desirable (or urgent) it may be to educate people towards this standard. If someone were to contract HIV as a result of unsafe sex practices – even today, some years after the sexual means of transmission have been scientifically determined – it may be unfair to say that it is that person's 'fault' for failing to take precautions. If one has not been properly educated to begin with, and especially if one consented to the sexual activity that led to infection under false pretence, it is difficult to see how one can be found at 'fault'.

Would it then be the 'fault' of the person from whom one contracted HIV? Certainly not if that person also had not been properly educated and had no reason to suspect infection. If, however, the person did have reason to think this and knowingly concealed it, I think we can say with some authority that he or she is morally blameworthy for failing to make this disclosure.

But let us be clear about wherein this fault or blameworthiness would reside. Certainly this person would be *causally* responsible for communicating HIV, in the sense that its development in another person could be traced back in a causal chain to some sexual involvement with him or her. But *causal* responsibility is not enough for *moral* responsibility. If I die from complications following the amputation of my leg, the surgeon who did the amputation would be part of the causal chain that led to my death, but would not necessarily be at fault. Moral fault requires something more than causal responsibility, and this something more may be difficult to pin down.

According to the liberal approach advocated in this paper, moral responsibility with respect to sexual ethics and AIDS is to be decided with reference to informed consent. I am at fault, and morally responsible (irresponsible), if I fail to give you information about my history or condition that would be germane to your decision (approximately, the decision of a reasonable person) to consent to sexual involvement with me. If, however, I have so informed you, and in light of this knowledge you give your consent, I am not, according to this approach, morally at fault if as a result of our sexual activity you become infected and subsequently go on to develop AIDS. The involvement would have been sanctioned by the fact of your informed consent. The requirement that consent be informed does not guarantee that what we choose will always turn out well, and certainly not that we will always choose wisely.

SOCIAL POLICY CONSIDERATIONS

The discussion of blameworthiness raises important questions about social policy in connection with the sexual transmission of HIV, this being a matter in which the state has considerable interest. There has been much discussion about legal rights and duties centred around the case of someone knowingly exposing others to HIV infection. Cases of this sort, in my view, have received exaggerated media attention, which moreover has often been coded in such a way as to feed or fuel the general hysteria and prejudice evident in our society towards people living with AIDS. For example, a headline in Halifax's *Chronicle-Herald* (19 September 1988), boldly emblazoned in blood red – 'AIDS fiend strikes again' – communicates a message that exceeds the requirements of mere reporting. That said, there is a legitimate issue here, which, although too complex to be done justice in a paper focused mainly on interpersonal ethics, is not altogether outside the scope of the argument I have advanced.[22]

Two cases, both of which were eventually handled through the Criminal Code, should serve to frame the issue. The first, the subject of the headline cited above, is the case of Scott Wentzell of Halifax, who had unprotected sexual intercourse with a woman who subsequently went on to become HIV-positive.[23] Having received counselling, he knew about the danger of infecting others, and yet neither took precautions nor informed the woman of the considerable risk she was taking on. Moreover, the woman was pregnant at the time (and quite likely to pass the infection to her baby), and there is some evidence that Wentzell knew she was pregnant. He was charged and pleaded guilty to criminal negligence causing bodily harm (section 204 of the Criminal Code).

The second case concerns Gordon Summers of Calgary.[24] The circumstances were much the same as in the Wentzell case, except that at least five people were involved over a two-year period, and Summers continued having unprotected sex even after he had learned that one of the persons with whom he had been sexually involved had gone on to become HIV-positive. Initially he was charged with aggravated assault but, after two of the women refused to testify against him, this was reduced to the lesser charge of committing a common nuisance by endangering the lives and health of the public, contrary to section 180 of the Criminal Code. Summers also pleaded guilty.

In my view, the wisdom of using the Criminal Code (and especially of using even more coercive instruments, such as quarantine) in cases such as these is open to debate.[25] Assuming for the purpose of argument the appropriateness of coercive measures, however, I have concerns about how coercion might be brought to bear. In these two cases, the courts focused on the fact that the individuals charged failed to practise safer sex knowing that in so doing they were exposing their partners to serious risk. From a liberal point of view, this is to put the emphasis in the wrong place. Certainly their failure to practise safer sex was reprehensible, but even more so was the fact that they did so while concealing information material to their partners' informed consent to be sexually involved with them.

Had the circumstances of these cases been different (for example, had those charged used reasonable precautions), it is possible that the consent issue might have been brought to the fore, but as it stands the implication seems to be that for someone who is HIV-infectious, practising safer sex is enough by way of discharging their duty toward sexual partners. This much is indeed important, but I submit that there is also and even more crucially a duty to inform sexual partners of one's HIV status insofar as this might have a bearing on their consent to sexual activity. Even if safer sex is being practised (intercourse with a condom, for example), and the risk therefore is low, the choice to take this risk belongs to the one who must bear its consequences.

Emphasizing choice in such matters, however, raises questions as to what extent the state should protect people from making choices that, although perhaps informed, are thought imprudent and harmful. For example, would informing a prospective partner that one is HIV-infectious be the basis of an acceptable defence against such charges, even in the extreme case where one's partner consents to unprotected intercourse? Not to recognize such a defence, it seems to me, would offend against liberty in two important ways. In the first place, it would offend against the principle that properly informed adults ought to be permitted to choose risks that might seem manifestly foolish to others, and moreover that in freely doing so they take upon themselves responsibility for any injury they may suffer (*volenti non fit injuria*).

In the second place, the absence of such a defence would in effect *legally require* people who know themselves to be HIV-positive to practise safer sex, and this would constitute a grave offence against individual privacy and liberty. To be sure, this would not be much of a burden, and probably the vast majority of people who know themselves to be HIV-infectious practise safer sex out of moral obligation anyway, but it would be an indignity to be in effect required to do so by law. Moreover, there being some risk even in safer sex, one can imagine how a one-sided and overzealous emphasis on prevention of harm might lead to a state of affairs in which HIV-infectious persons would be altogether prohibited from sexual activity with others, consenting or not.

Liberty, however, is not an absolute value, and must be balanced against other important values. In principle, at least, everyone will agree that it is legitimate in certain circumstances for the state to interfere with liberty in order to maintain or promote some other important value. Perhaps, it might be argued, it is in fact necessary to do so in order to curtail the spread of AIDS throughout our society.

There is reason to doubt that coercive measures would indeed further this important objective, but even granting the premise it could be argued that other, less liberty-offending means could do the job just as well as could legally requiring (in effect) people who know themselves to be HIV-positive to practise safer sex. Placing the emphasis differently, the state instead could require them to inform sexual partners of their HIV status. This would be more respectful of liberty, and, I believe, would lead to more or less the same outcome, as very few people, it can be presumed, would choose to have unsafe sex with people known by them to be HIV-infectious (and very few people who know themselves to be HIV-infectious would not be practising safer sex).

NOTES

[1]This association is especially dubious when, as often happens, it is interpreted causally. Homosexuality is no more a cause of AIDS than is heterosexuality (or haemophilia).

[2]For an excellent critical analysis of the moralizing approach to AIDS, see Eric Matthews, 'AIDS and Sexual Morality', *Bioethics* 2, 2 (1988): 118-28.

[3]For a more detailed discussion of the liberal approach to sexual ethics as contrasted with other points of view, see Russell Vannoy, *Sex Without Love: A Philosophical Exploration* (Buffalo: Prometheus Books, 1980), especially pp. 120-5.

[4]Thinking about sexual ethics in terms of consent is a relatively recent development, and goes hand in hand with the increased valuing of individual autonomy in our society in recent years (especially evident when one examines the history of informed consent in the health-care context). In an excellent historical analysis of sexual ethics, Margaret Farley writes: 'contemporary efforts to develop a new sexual ethic are to a great extent based on new interpretations not only of human sexuality but of the human person. Thus, for example, new emphases on the element of human freedom in the complex structure of the person give rise to norms for sexual behavior that place greater emphasis on the need for the free consent of both sexual partners' (*Bibliography of Bioethics*, s.v. 'sexual ethics').

[5]A comprehensive philosophical discussion of informed consent is given in Ruth R. Faden and Tom L. Beauchamp, *A History and Theory of Informed Consent* (New York: Oxford University Press, 1986). The term 'informed consent' is less than ideal insofar as it suggests a certain passivity whereby one simply responds to options laid out and initiated by another. What I have in mind might better be captured by the phrase 'informed choice', which is a more empowering term.

[6]HIV stands for 'human immunodeficiency virus', which is generally believed to cause AIDS. People who are HIV-positive, even if they do not have AIDS, are believed to be capable of transmitting the virus to others.

[7]Canadian AIDS Society, *Safer Sex Guidelines: A Resource Document for Educators and Counsellors*, Ottawa, March 1988.

[8]Ibid., p. 6.

[9]Ibid.

[10]See Faden and Beauchamp, pp. 30-4.

[11]This standard was first introduced into Canadian law with reference to medical negligence in the *Reibl v. Hughes* case. A concise summary of this case and how this standard came to be articulated is given in Gilbert Sharpe, *The Law and Medicine in Canada*, 2nd ed. (Toronto: Butterworths, 1987), especially pp. 42-55.

This standard is not without difficulties. Are we to believe that the 'reasonable person' is invariant across boundaries of gender, culture, and social class? What about the specific context in light of which a particular person might give or fail to give consent? This line of questioning argues in favour of what is called a 'subjective standard' of disclosure, according to which disclosure should be individually tailored to specific contexts; e.g., what would be germane to the consent of *this particular person in this particular set of circumstances, etc.*

[12]The concept of 'maternal risk' is very important for analysing disclosure requirements. In the precedent-setting *Reibl v. Hughes* case, Justice Laskin specified that 'if a certain risk is a mere possibility which ordinarily need not be disclosed, yet if

its occurrence carries serious consequences . . . it should be regarded as a material risk requiring disclosure' (quoted in Gilbert Sharpe, p. 44). Following this line of thinking, it is clear that the risk even of sexual activity deemed low-risk according to *Guidelines* would be material to a reasonable person's informed consent.

[13]It may well be that, according to other norms – for example, that one should be open about one's past in a relationship – she is entitled to this information, but I am restricting myself to explicitly liberal norms.

[14]Aristotle, *Nichomachean Ethics*, 2nd ed., trans. H. Rackham (London: Harvard University Press, 1934), I. iii. 4.

[15]Quoted in Judith Haines, 'V International Conference on AIDS', *The Canadian Nurse* 85, 7 (August 1989): 21.

[16]Leslie Baxter and William Wilmot, 'Taboo Topics in Close Relationships', *Journal of Social and Personal Relationships* 2 (1985): 253–69.

[17]'The Crisis of Communicating in Relationships: Confronting the Threat of AIDS', *AIDS & Public Policy Journal* 4, 1: 18. Gender-specific differences about information-acquiring strategies in sexual relationships are also reported in Leslie Baxter and William Wilmot, 'Secret Tests: Social Strategies for Acquiring Information About the State of the Relationship', *Human Communication Research* 11, 2 (Winter 1984): 197.

[18]*Guidelines*, 34-6.

[19]Safer sex does substantially reduce risks, but breakage and improper use of condoms (10 to 15 per cent failure rate in contraception) are also a reality. See Cornelius Rietmeijer et al., 'Condoms as Physical and Chemical Barriers Against Human Immunodeficiency Virus', *Journal of the American Medical Association* 259, 12 (March 1989): 1851–3. Rietmeijer et al. present evidence suggesting that supplementary use of a spermicide or viricide is to some degree effective as a backup in instances of condom failure, but research in this area is still inconclusive. The authors of *Guidelines* explicitly state that nonoxynol-9, the only chemical barrier sufficiently tested at this time to warrant their recommendation, 'should not be used for rectal sex' (p. 21). The unreliability of condom use as a means of preventing transmission (however small) has led some to view condom use as a '*secondary* strategy' for risk minimization. See James Goedert, 'What is Safe Sex?', *New England Journal of Medicine* 316, 21: 1340.

[20]Screening strategies are compared with safer sex by Norman Hearst and Stephen Hulley, who argue that in the American heterosexual population screening strategies may be more effective than the practice of safer sex by way of risk minimization ('Preventing the Heterosexual Spread of AIDS: Are We Giving Our Patients the Best Advice?', *Journal of the American Medical Association* 259, 16 : 2428–32).

[21]For statistics (alarming) about the practice of safer sex among young people, see *Canada Youth & AIDS Study*, Social Program Evaluation Group, Queen's University (Ottawa: Health and Welfare Canada, 1988), especially pp. 104–5.

[22]For a more detailed consideration of the legal issues only superficially touched on here, see Bernard Dickens, 'Legal Rights and Duties in the AIDS Epidemic', *Science* 239 (5 Feb. 1988): 580–6.

[23]*R. v. Scott Wentzell*, Preliminary Hearing, Magisterial District of Nova Scotia, Kennedy J., 18 Jan. 1989.

[24]Q.B. Alta., 11289, 10 Aug. 1989, Dinkel J. (unreported).

[25]A good case against coercive measures is given by Richard Mohr, *Gays/Justice: A Study of Ethics, Society, and Law* (New York: Columbia University Press, 1988), and by David Mayo in 'AIDS, Quarantines, and Noncompliant Positives', in Christine Pierce and Donald VanDeVeer, eds, *AIDS, Ethics and Public Policy* (Belmont, CA: Wadsworth, 1988), 113–23.

HEALTH-CARE WORKERS' OCCUPATIONAL EXPOSURE TO HIV: OBLIGATIONS AND ENTITLEMENTS

BENJAMIN FREEDMAN

> From the contagion of the world's slow stain
> He is secure . . .
> Percy Bysshe Shelley, *Adonais*

THE DUTY TO TREAT[1]

Introduction

The human immunodeficiency virus (HIV) is more than a pathogen: it is a complicated bundle of paradox and contradiction. It is a leading public health problem, caused by the most private of activities. It bears plague, the ancient scourge of humanity, into a modern era that thought itself, in the privileged West, free of epidemic; and its rapid spread is facilitated by the modern ill of intravenous drug abuse and the complicated technological achievement of world-wide integration through transportation. It wreaks its damage by appropriating to its own deadly use the body's basic defence mechanism against disease.

The ethical paradoxes associated with HIV are no less notable. In this paper I concentrate upon one issue: the health-care worker's (and, especially, the physician's) obligation to treat patients infectious for HIV. (I shall speak of 'HIV-infectious' patients, rather than of those who are 'HIV-infected' or 'HIV-positive', to emphasize the doctor's concern with contagion. Patients need not be HIV-positive to be contagious; prior to seroconversion,[2] the infected person is clearly contagious.[3] In addition, growing experience with the disease suggests that infected patients vary in infectiousness as the disease runs its course.)[4]

The paradoxes are numerous. For example, a profession instituted to care for the ill ponders whether it has a duty to care for the desperately ill person with AIDS. A response is mounted by several authors who have reached the right conclusion – that there is a duty to treat – for what seem to me the wrong reasons. It is important to explore this paradox, for it has implications for our understanding of medicine's past traditions, present practices, and future challenges. In doing that, a final paradox needs to be faced: for all the ink that has been spilled regarding the duty to care for the HIV-infectious, almost nothing has been said of the privileges accompanying that duty.

Health-care workers' risk of occupational acquisition of HIV infection has been reviewed in detail,[5] and is the subject of ongoing prospective and retrospective study in Canada and elsewhere.[6] Several salient points emerge:

The risk can be delineated, and is largely confined to those exposed to HIV-infectious blood by needlestick injury or through a splash onto an open wound or a mucous membrane.

The risk can be reduced, by use of barrier precautions limiting such exposure.[7]

The risk is small. Even those exposed are very unlikely to become infected; perhaps one in two hundred needlestick exposures from known HIV carriers will seroconvert.[8]

The risk is real. Even presuming effective use of uniform blood and body-fluid barrier precautions, some exposures will occur, and a few of those exposed will seroconvert and go on to develop AIDS.

When the possibility of occupational AIDS risk was first perceived in North America, a number of physicians and some medical organizations declared that this new threat modified and limited the physician's obligation to his or her patients. Such public statements quickly grew scarce, in the face of an opposing stance adopted by bodies including state licensure boards, human–rights commissions, and, ultimately, the American Medical Association[9] (followed, after a decent delay, by the Canadian Medical Association).[10] The public consensus that there is an enforceable professional duty on the part of doctors to treat HIV-infectious patients was bolstered by several articles (which I shall discuss below) describing the ethical underpinnings of this duty. Yet some of the arguments most commonly appealed to in establishing the duty are demonstrably weak, and ethicists above all need to concern themselves with the validity of the arguments employed as well as with their conclusion.

'This Was Part of the Deal'. Within our fragmented ethical world, the most common form of duty that we understand is self-imposed: the duty to keep promises, to fulfil contracts and commitments.[11] It is therefore not surprising

to hear that doctors have a duty to treat the infectious because that risk is an unwelcome but unavoidable part of the deal a person makes in entering the practice of medicine. The argument appears in several versions, each one problematic in its own way.

Raanan Gillon argues that *individual* physicians have accepted this risk: 'As health care professionals we accept obligations to treat our patients even when this entails what might be called real risks.'[12] This argument makes sense when addressed to students of medicine and nursing today, for it is now established that there is an occupational HIV risk out of which trainees and practitioners may not contract. But this cannot be said of persons who chose, trained, and established a practice without knowing that this risk loomed over the horizon. Would they have chosen medicine, knowing that this risk would occur? It is impossible to say, although the severe drop in medical-school applications that the United States is now experiencing may suggest that they would not. (Because of the high rate of infection in the US relative to other Western nations, including Canada, American reaction is often seen as a harbinger of trends that may crop up elsewhere.) At any rate, what doctors *would* have done *had* they known is irrelevant. They did not in fact know, and so did not in fact agree to undergo this risk.

While HIV occupational risk was not an *explicit* part of the undertaking, however, some will suggest it is implicitly incorporated within the broad category of risk to which persons have agreed. The risk to health-care workers of dying from occupationally induced hepatitis B remains much greater than HIV risk.[13] If individuals accept equivalent or greater risks, as part of the implied contract of employment as a physician, why not subsume HIV risk in this way? One illustration of the seemingly inconsistent reactions a person may have to different risks was related to me by Dr Sheldon Landesman, describing a question raised at an AIDS symposium. The questioner, a surgeon who was also a volunteer fireman, was asking about the risk of infection from providing mouth-to-mouth resuscitation to a burn victim. Even while responding to the question, Landesman expressed bemusement at concern over a small risk of contagion on the part of someone who voluntarily spends his spare time racing into burning buildings![14]

This last example itself demonstrates a problem with the argument. Individuals within our society are, in general, entitled to choose the form and level of risk they will undergo; it is the chief object of both criminal and regulatory law to ensure that this principle be respected. There is, moreover, no definitive, 'rational' response to risk that can be imposed – for example, when someone who has already accepted the risk of hepatitis B is told that it is irrational for him to reject the increment of HIV risk As Daniel Kahneman and Amos Tversky have shown,[15] ideas of rationality and even of logical consistency (e.g., the transitivity of choices) are themselves controversial as applied to judgements of risk; in part, because our models of rationality impose dubious boundary conditions like atemporality. Clearly, too, the manner of death by AIDS, medically and socially, bears with it a particular dread that does not necessarily attach to other occupational risks.

The American Medical Association has adopted still a third version of the argument that 'this risk was part of the deal'. In its view, a duty to treat the HIV-infectious flows from a historically accepted principle of medical ethics: 'When an epidemic prevails, a physician must continue his own labors without regard to the risk to his own health.'[16] By this account, while the duty to treat need not have been an explicit or implicit individual undertaking, it is a long-standing *communal* undertaking on the part of the profession, which can be imputed to individual members as well.[17]

To its credit, the AMA has maintained this stance from its very beginnings; the above-quoted statement was first employed in the AMA's original code of ethics, adopted in 1847. Yet it did not then, nor does it now, have the power of attorney on behalf of every physician, such that it could bind him or her to a contract the AMA signs.

The AMA may claim to be *expressing*, rather than *establishing*, a professional obligation. It may claim, that is, that the duty to stand by patients at times of epidemic has always been acknowledged by physicians, and that its statement merely codified this obligation. Recent historical research into physicians' behaviour in times of epidemic, however, undertaken specifically in a search for guidance by precedent, reveals a very mixed picture.[18] While many physicians stayed to treat patients, many others, including prominent and respected members of the profession, fled. While some accounts criticize those who fled for unethical conduct, other accounts find those who stayed guilty of the same charge – because, for example, they placed their other patients at risk of infection. To ground a professional obligation within practice, that practice needs to be widespread if not actually uniform, and self-consciously adopted with specifically ethical motivation. The historical record of physicians faced with epidemic disease supports neither requirement.

'We Expect More From Physicians'. A second set of arguments very commonly offered as grounding an obligation to treat the infectious revolves around a form of *noblesse oblige*. By this account, physicians may justifiably be held to a higher standard of moral conduct than others, a higher standard that includes a degree of self-sacrifice on behalf of the welfare of patients.

Abigail Zuger and Steven Miles argue, for example, that the duty to care for the infectious patient is not a result of contract ('this is part of the deal') nor of a patient's right to be treated, but is rather an expression of professional virtue.[19] Ethics measures character as well as conduct, and the good physician may be expected to adhere to high standards of courage, integrity, and loyalty to the patient. These virtues are tested, and gain correspondingly in importance, when treating patients in a time of epidemic. Gillon makes a similar point when he writes to and of his fellow physicians, 'We still commit ourselves to the characteristic medical obligation to benefit our patients.'[20] And Edmund Pellegrino, who has been prominent among those writing of the unique ethical features of medicine, argues that a duty to treat HIV-infectious patients follows from medicine's effacement of self-interest on the part of its practitioners, a step that is based upon the nature of professional commitment to the ill person; the public, non-proprietary character of medical knowledge; and the public avowal of professional responsibility expressed in the oath taken by those entering the profession.[21]

I have considerable sympathy for this stance.[22] Unlike the previous argument, maintaining that HIV risk was already accepted by professionals, this view holds that special ethical standards uniquely appropriate to and incumbent upon the medical profession include a duty to undergo the risk in treating infectious patients. Ultimately, I believe there *is* a special – and, in some respects, higher – ethical standard to which medical practitioners must be held. Nonetheless, I find these arguments unconvincing in the specific context of a duty to treat the infectious.

First, in response to Miles and Zuger, it may be said that it is patients themselves who have insisted upon respecting rights and contracts in medical practice, most notably through 'consumer' demands for patient autonomy and the right to consent, and (notoriously) in malpractice litigation. A physician may be excused for believing that the insistence by laypersons on rights has poisoned the warm, trusting soil within which an ethic of virtue must grow. I repeat: I do not agree with this view; but I have sympathy for the practitioner who feels caught in a catch-22, within which the ethical rules are always employed to his detriment. Connected is the perception by physicians that the privileges granted to the profession are ever decreasing: 'If we are so "*obligé*", where is the "*noblesse*"'?

These views are inadequate for another reason: they are not comprehensive. Occupational risk of HIV is shared across professional lines, by dentists, nurses, and blood technicians, as well as by physicians and surgeons. They all bear the risk, and, I believe, they all bear the same ethical duty. Yet if that is true, the ethical duty surely cannot be based in an ethic unique to the medical profession. Indeed, some physicians may state that while they accept the risk on their own behalf, they cannot expose their spouses to it, in the event of infection from an unnoticed occupational exposure. The claim would probably be disingenuous – but it is not *necessarily* so. Is there another approach to this issue that avoids these problems while providing a comprehensive basis for the duty to treat the infectious?

The Results of Refusal to Care

A thought experiment will clarify the proper basis for this duty to treat the infectious. Imagine that the profession decides to the contrary, that there is *no* such duty. Every practitioner is left free to refuse to care for HIV-infectious patients, and this exclusionary decision is no cause for professional discipline or even for adverse comment from the leaders of the profession. What would be the predictable results of this policy?

Obviously, a number of practitioners would be tempted to establish an 'AIDS-free' practice. It is impossible to estimate what proportion of practitioners would succumb to this temptation. Even under present circumstances, some have stated publicly that they exclude HIV-infectious patients, and many more have said this *sotto voce*. To these would be added, within our hypothetical scenario, those deterred to date solely by fear of professional discipline (e.g., loss of hospital privileges), or the more informal sanction of adverse public comment and moral criticism. For that matter, there is, presumably, a cohort that does not discriminate against the HIV-infectious for reasons of conscience, and some of these, within our scenario, would find that – contrary to what they had believed – there is no *moral* necessity to continue to subject themselves to this unwanted risk.

My guess, for what it is worth, is that initially a significant but not overwhelming proportion of non-hospital-based practitioners would opt for an 'AIDS-free' practice; and that this proportion might rise over time. I would guess further that the distribution of refusers would not be geographically uniform, so that there would be some regions of low population density where *most* local practitioners would opt to refuse. The primary means that these refusers will have to exclude the HIV-infectious will be through serum screening, of all patients or of those patients who seem likely to be at risk of infection.

What then would follow? Fear within the community at large would be bolstered and legitimated. The facts are, as we have seen, that the risk of health-care occupational transmission of HIV is small and controllable, but that permitting physicians to purport to exclude the HIV-infectious would send the opposite signals: that anyone dealing with a person with AIDS is at risk; that HIV risk is unavoidable; and that those persons who know the most about this – doctors themselves – are worried. An important moral message is sent as well: that HIV status is an acceptable basis for depriving persons of rights and services.

These messages of panic and discrimination are in themselves deeply worrying, but worse is to come. The refusing practitioner is worried about infectiousness, but his or her only reliable evidence for that will be serum-negative status. Yet as we know, there is an HIV 'window-period' between a person's acquiring the infection and seroconverting. The 'window period' is commonly two to three months, but can be as long as a year.[23] Throughout that period, the person is at least as infectious as one who has seroconverted.

It is for this reason that I have referred to the 'AIDS-free' practice in quotation marks. Even with universal and regularly repeated screening of all patients, no practitioner could honestly make that claim. There is one way of ensuring that a person with negative serum status is not infected – by ascertaining that he or she has not engaged in any HIV-risky behaviour for the previous twelve months – but this path is unfortunately not available to the refuser. Those who are at risk will, predictably, lie to their refusing physician about their behaviour in order to retain his or her services. Without justifying the lie, I must admit that under these circumstances I would find it hard to criticize the liar.

Two further circumstances will ensue. Practitioners who believe they have excluded the risk of occupational HIV infection may be lulled into a false sense of security, and omit onerous and expensive adherence to uniform barrier precautions, thus putting themselves at higher risk of infection. And, as a corollary to Gresham's Law in economics (good money drives out bad), practitioners who claim – falsely – to have 'AIDS-free' practices will reap the benefit of their falsehood, by adding to their practices credulous and panicked patients, to the detriment of their more scrupulous colleagues.

I have saved for the last those consequences that are, in my judgement, the most worrisome and ethically troubling. Those excluding patients known or thought to be HIV-infectious externalize their risk to those colleagues who refuse to practice this discrimination, resulting in an unjustified concentration of risk. This would be deeply unfair.

Finally, legitimate efforts to test patients for HIV status, and to exchange this information in health-care settings, would be crippled. In its day, syphilis was known as the 'great impostor', a disease whose effects could mimic the symptoms of a myriad of ailments, confounding differential diagnosis. Clearly, HIV disease is taking on that grim role today, and exclusion of HIV may become the first step in diagnosis for a large proportion of presenting patients.[24] In the interests of the responsible provision of health care, it will become absolutely essential that HIV status be information shared among providers, no less than with any other systemic disease.

At some point, discussions of AIDS and confidentiality will need to come to terms with this medical and ethical imperative. In the context of a policy that permits physicians to refuse to care for the HIV-infectious with impunity, however, it will be quite impossible to elicit and share this information honestly. Patients who know they are or might be infected will have a powerful motivation for concealment, for fear of losing access to health care. Many such patients will be aided in their efforts to conceal or evade by those practitioners who know of their HIV status, but are equally concerned that their patients not lose access to the services of others. If a practitioner may refuse to treat someone who is HIV-infectious, doctors may refuse to tell dentists, pulmonary specialists may refuse to tell surgeons, house staff may refuse to tell nurses. Discrimination breeds concealment, and the free exchange of information is essential to modern team approaches to health-care delivery. That approach requires discretion and confidentiality of the patient–team relationship, not simply of the traditional patient–doctor dyad.[25]

The Duty to Treat: Conclusion

I have argued that the professional duty to treat the HIV-infectious is not grounded upon a prior agreement to undergo this risk. From this point on, however, it clearly is: anyone entering a health-care profession now must realize that 'this is part of the deal'. The duty is not based upon any extraordinary moral obligations incumbent upon physicians – even though I believe such obligations do indeed exist. It is, rather, based upon a realistic appreciation of how harmful the results would be were such discrimination to be permitted, as well as an elementary concern for fairness: that discriminators not reap the rewards of their fear and dissimulation, and that non-discriminators not be subjected to added risk in picking up the slack left by their colleagues.

Sooner or later, in discussions of ethics and AIDS, someone is bound to argue against a supposed privilege or right of AIDS patients by asking why this disease is so special. Why establish a duty to treat persons infectious with HIV, for example, when in general a physician is an autonomous professional, free to limit practice however he or she chooses? Therein lies the final paradox. In principle I agree that HIV should be treated exactly on a par with any relevantly similar pathogen; yet it is only with AIDS patients that the question of discrimination arises. We search the current literature in vain for discussions of the right to refuse to treat those infectious with hepatitis, those terminally ill with disseminated cancer, those who are ungrateful or distasteful. AIDS belongs within the ordinary continuum of human ailments; but it will take extraordinary attention on the part of society in general and the health-care community in particular before we are prepared to admit that.

THE LIMITS OF RISK AND COMPENSATION[26]

In defining a territory, we describe its boundaries. Even so, in delineating a moral duty of health professionals to treat patients in spite of risk of infection, we must be prepared to describe its limits. At what level would the danger of infection be so extreme that the moral duty to treat would be abrogated? In a logical sense, until we can define the *limit* of the duty, we have failed to define the duty itself; and in a practical sense, without defining the limit of the duty, we cannot know whether it has any current application. As a society, though, we have difficulty in dealing rationally with risk assessment; and the issue of occupational risk in particular has received little serious academic attention. The following comments are intended simply to highlight some of the complexities that require examination.

Occupations and Risk

Most discussions of the duty to treat have ignored the essential question of the relationship between obligation and risk. One exception is a statement on

AIDS of the American Nurses' Association that posits a duty to treat the infectious patient when the value of the care supplied outweighs the risk to the nurse, provided that the danger 'does not represent more than minimal risk to the health care provider.'[27] The ANA failed, however, to define what it meant by 'minimal risk', or to quantify that risk. And so, while we know that the risk faced by the nurse when that statement was adopted (13 Nov. 1986) fell below the threshold value of minimal risk, since the ANA at that time affirmed a duty to treat, we cannot extrapolate from that to a contemporary duty, if the current risk is greater.

Indeed it *is* greater, for the risk to a health-care worker is a function of the rate at which exposures to infected blood (primarily, via needlestick injuries) cause infection in the injured party, *and of the proportion of patients who are themselves infected.* Although, as noted above, the former rate is low – roughly one in two hundred incidents leads to infection – the latter rate (the proportion of the hospital population infected with HIV) is much higher than was the case in 1986, and is continuing to increase. Has the benchmark of ethically obligatory risk established by the ANA already been passed?

There is another problem with the 'minimal risk' level. This level is a familiar benchmark in the ethics of human research, where it is understood to represent the level of risk ordinarily encountered in *everyday life.*[28] Some feel this to be the appropriate level for occupational risk as well; for example, a report from the Health Advocacy Unit of the City of Toronto has maintained that 'workers should not be exposed to greater health risks than the general public'.[29] Even there, though, the statement is avowedly one of a distant ideal; the more common feeling is that 'pursuing one's trade will almost inevitably bring a peculiar set of risks, ... allowably ... greater than for non-occupational purposes'.[30] This feeling has been particularly strong among health-care workers with respect to an occupational risk of infection, perhaps because they are self-selected into what Rowe has called 'value groups', people who share a common attitude towards, or valuation of, risk.[31]

In general, our individual tolerance of risk is raised when the risk is understood, predictable, and, especially, under our control[32] – in short, voluntary. The point seems intuitive: we are more comfortable with the consequences of our own actions – and mistakes – than with hazards imposed upon us. Another factor causing a voluntary/involuntary risk disparity was pointed out by Mark Sagoff: *resentment* when we are exposed to risk against our will, and thus treated as the means to another's end.[33]

It would seem that risk imposed occupationally is in several respects *voluntarily* undergone; hence, towards the higher end of acceptable risk.[34] The contrary claim has it that whenever a worker undergoes an occupational risk, he or she has been coerced into that choice under economic pressure;[35] but coercion in that (very extended) sense is of limited ethical significance. Even the weakest – most grudging and most limited – acceptance of a concept of paid labour implies the existence of some form of acceptable trade-off of risk for wages. This is true even if the job carries with it no more risk than does everyday life itself; for jobs, unlike everyday life, carry with them risks borne on specific account of the wage benefit, rather than other forms of benefit.

The *particular instances of risk* to which one is subjected on the job (e.g., video-terminal radiation when working on a computer) would not be accepted in everyday life. Magnitude is not the issue: an employee might refuse to work with a VDT, yet play video games for hours on end, though the latter involves more radiation. One may choose radiation for game enjoyment, not for dollars; contrariwise, those who choose to work with VDTs do so for money, not for the love of little green luminous letters.

At a first level, then, we may speak of some level of risk that comes with the job itself; payment for both is one package deal. At some point, though, occupational risk becomes great enough that a special wage premium ought to be paid.

Risk Premiums

Some points potentially relevant to health-care workers and HIV emerge from a US review of the literature that confirmed the existence of a risk-wage trade-off in that country.[36] The authors noticed that while some employees (e.g., skilled workers with explosives) are well-reimbursed on account of attendant risk, others are in quite risky occupations but ill-paid nonetheless. (The data on risk are full of surprises: included among the relatively high-risk occupations without adequate compensation are bartenders, cocktail waitresses, and door-to-door salesmen. I say this with bemusement, but no intended irony.)

The authors propose a distinction between two sorts of labour markets. In the *primary* labour market, jobs are characterized by good income, job security, unionization, and benefits – and a genuine risk premium that may be discerned within wages. For those in the *secondary* labour market – those who work without the advantages noted above, those who are unskilled, and those who work on a part-time basis – the risk premium is smaller or absent. One reason for the disparity may be the greater mobility and lower employment in the primary labour market. Also, primary-market workers have access to more information than do the others; they are commonly more educated, and in any event have access to information through unions and professional bodies.

Other anomalies were also noted. For example, the risk premium seems to operate in compensation for accidents (especially those that result in fatalities) much more strongly than for work-related sickness. This may well be another manifestation of differentials in available information. The authors find, suggestively, that there is very little if any risk premium on behalf of work-related life-style factors, although these undoubtedly are important determinants of morbidity.

Should such a premium be paid to health-care workers because of the occupational risk of HIV? In Canada at present the risks are so low that this would be an exaggerated response. These risks are not, however, geographically even, and may shift over time. I will conclude with a number of points emerging from the above:

1. Any risk premium ought to be tied to the genuine occupational risk undergone. These risks are only weakly determined by occupational title (doctor, nurse, etc.). They are more strongly influenced by the *functions* performed, and are increased, for example, for emergency-room personnel (because of emergency-room working conditions as well as the variety of problems posed and interventions attempted), or those working in certain kinds of surgical theatres (e.g., obstetric, oral, orthopaedic). And they are *most* strongly influenced by the nature of the population served, and its rate of infection.

2. Risk premiums depend upon accurate risk information. This should be relatively simple to obtain and deal with in the context of occupational HIV transmission, an area that has been the subject of intensive surveillance and prospective study. (Because of its simple causal route of transmission, occupational HIV is much more like a common 'occupational accident' – e.g., in construction – than common 'occupational illness' caused by long-term, low-level, chronic exposures.)

3. Risk premiums have the potential to reflect job, sex, and race discrimination. If HIV-risk premiums were to follow the pattern discerned within other contexts – and there is absolutely no reason to suppose the contrary – physicians will receive near-adequate reimbursement, unionized nurses something approaching that, and others little or none. These 'others' are all within the vulnerable 'secondary' labour market, and include nursing assistants and practical nurses, dental hygienists, and orderlies – classes of occupation at a level of occupational risk equivalent to that faced by physicians and nurses. Within these occupations, of course, women and disadvantaged minorities overwhelmingly predominate. This is a group with few choices: occupational risk is for them, therefore, relatively *in*voluntary, and the argument for compensation is correspondingly strengthened.

As with the duty to treat the HIV-infectious, here again I would point to the importance of equity and of fellow-feeling among health-care workers. Precisely because this is an epidemic that tends to tear us apart as a society, it presents us with the opportunity to affirm the contrary values of solidarity.

Occupational Risk: Conclusion

At the time of writing, I have yet to encounter any other discussion, written or oral, of risk premiums for those treating patients infectious for HIV. Why not? In one sense, the reason is obvious: by my own admission, the risk at present is much too low to justify hazard pay. The discussion is therefore premature; speculation is alarmist.

I am not satisfied with this response, however. It is, after all, the job of academics and policy analysts to *anticipate* issues before they arise. The ethical case for risk premiums falls within responsible extrapolation, for in some regions it will certainly arise. Already, many hospitals in the New York metropolitan region report that 5 per cent of their admissions are infected with HIV; for some, the figures are much higher.

Canadian figures are incomparably lower at present, and it is to be hoped that they will never approach those levels. We do not, however, *know* that New York levels have peaked, nor where Canadian levels will peak. The present validated facts of HIV are grim enough, some may feel. For them, speculation concerning what could happen is out of place, even irresponsible.

I reject this view. In our reluctance to borrow trouble by planning ahead, we defeat our own purpose: we intensify the aura of crisis surrounding society's reaction to HIV. My own belief is that such speculation – clearly identified as such – is needed. Rather than being alarmist, such speculation may send a signal that the future holds nothing so awful that we cannot plan for it in a sensible fashion.

NOTES

[1] The first section of this paper appeared in slightly altered form in *Canadian Family Physician* under the title 'Is There a Duty To Provide Medical Care to HIV-Infectious Patients? Facts, Fallacies, Fairness, and the Future'. I am grateful to Dr Norbert Gilmore for his comments and assistance on this portion of the manuscript. Christine Overall suggested several useful suggestions, which I have incorporated. All errors and omissions are, however, my own.

[2] 'Seroconversion' refers to the production of antibodies specific to an infection. As this is being written, and as has been true since the discovery of HIV, the main means of detecting whether an individual has been infected is by testing his or her blood for the presence of antibodies, which represent an indirect but firm indication of exposure to the virus. A person in whose bloodstream HIV antibodies are detected is said to have 'seroconverted', or to be (through an elision) 'HIV-positive'. As discussed later in this paper, there is a delay – the so-called 'window period' – between infection and the body's recognition of infection evidenced by antibody production. Some persons with very advanced AIDS will lose seropositivity, as their immune system no longer has the ability to produce antibodies; in addition, in a very few cases, a person at the time of infection may already have so profoundly impaired an immune system (e.g., because of having taken immunosuppressive drugs) that antibodies are never produced at all. Research toward direct detection of the virus and, perhaps, gene amplification techniques may result in different standard means of viral detection and a shortened window period.

[3] J.W. Ward, S.D. Holmberg, J.R. Allen, *et al.*, 'Transmission of Human Immunodeficiency Virus (HIV) By Blood Transfusions Screened as Negative for HIV Antibody', *New England Journal of Medicine* 318, 8 (25 Feb. 1988): 473–8.

[4]R.M. Anderson and R.M. May, 'Epidemiological Parameters of HIV Transmission', *Nature* 333 (1988): 514-18; J. Albert, P. Olov Pehrson, S. Schulman, *et al.*, 'HIV Isolation and Antigen Detection in Infected Individuals and their Seronegative Sexual Partners', *AIDS* 2 (1988): 107-11.

[5]'Occupational Exposure to the Human Immunodeficiency Virus Among Health Care Workers in Canada', *Canadian Medical Association Journal* 140 (1 March 1989): 503-5.

[6]Ibid., n. 3; Ruthanne Marcus and the CDC Cooperative Needlestick Surveillance Group, 'Surveillance of Health Care Workers Exposed to Blood from Patients Infected with the Human Immunodeficiency Virus', *New England Journal of Medicine* 319, 17 (27 Oct. 1988): 1118-22.

[7]Federal Centre for AIDS, 'Recommendations for Prevention of HIV Transmission in Health-Care Settings', *Canada Diseases Weekly Report*, vol. I3S3 (Nov. 1987).

[8]Marcus *et al.*, n. 4.

[9]Benjamin Freedman, 'Health Professions, Codes, and the Right to Refuse to Treat HIV-Infectious Patients', in *AIDS: The Responsibilities of Health Practitioners*, special supplement to *Hastings Center Report* 8, 2 (April-May 1988): 20-5.

[10]'CMA Position: Acquired Immunodeficiency Syndrome', *Canadian Medical Association Journal* 140, (1 Jan. 1989): 64a.

[11]The most complete critique of contract as the denatured basis for liberal ethical thought that I know of is found in Michael Sandel, *Liberalism and the Limits of Justice* (New York: Cambridge University Press, 1982).

[12]Raanan Gillon, 'Refusal to Treat AIDS and HIV Positive Patients', *British Medical Journal* 294 (23 May 1987): 1332.

[13]'It is important to compare the observed risks to health care workers of HIV infection with the 6 percent to 30 percent risk of acquiring HBV [hepatitis B] infection after parenteral exposure to the blood of HBV infected patients' (James Allen, 'Health Care Workers and the Risk of HIV Transmission', in Hastings Center Supplement, n. 9).

[14]Sheldon Landesman, private communication; anecdote used by permission.

[15]Daniel Kahneman and Amos Tversky, 'The Psychology of Preferences', *Scientific American* 246, 1 (1982): 162.

[16]American Medical Association, Council on Ethical and Judicial Affairs, 'Ethical Issues Involved in the Growing AIDS Crisis', December 1987.

[17]Further questions concerning the relationship between codes of ethics and the behaviour of professionals, as well as the role of codes as reflecting behaviour or expressing ideals, are explored at length in Freedman, n. 9.

[18]Daniel M. Fox, 'The Politics of Physicians' Responsibility in Epidemics: A Note on History', in *AIDS: The Responsibilities of Health Professionals*, Hastings Center Supplement, n. 9.

[19]Abigail Zuger and Steven H. Miles, 'Physicians, AIDS, and Occupational Risk', *Journal of the American Medical Association* 258 (9 Oct. 1987): 1924-8.

[20]Gillon, n. 9.

[21]Edmund Pellegrino, 'Altruism, Self-interest, and Medical Ethics' (editorial) *Journal of the American Medical Association* 258, 14 (9 Oct. 1987): 1939-40.

[22]Benjamin Freedman, 'A Meta-ethics for Professional Morality', *Ethics* 89, 1 (1978).

[23]C. Pedersen, C.M. Nielsen, B.F. Vestergaard, et al., 'Temporal Relation of Antigenaemia and Loss of Antibodies to Core Antigens to Development of Clinical Disease in HIV Infection', *British Medical Journal* 295 (1987): 576-9.

[24]Norbert Gilmore, 'Patient Care for AIDS', *Transplantation/Implantation Today* 5 (September 1988): 47-50.

[25]This point is suggested by Norbert Gilmore's 'Protection of Sensitive Health Information in an Epidemic Situation: From the Doctor-Patient Dialogue to the Computer', presented at the World Health Organization Consultation on Health Legislation and Ethics in AIDS and HIV Infection, Oslo, 26 April 1988.

[26]This section builds upon, and in part quotes, my unpublished monograph 'Toward Consensus in Regulating Risks in Society: A Study of Issues and Methods', study paper prepared for the Protection of Life Project, Law Reform Commission of Canada, October 1983. I am grateful to the Commission and to my colleagues on that project (especially Edward Keyserlingk, director of the project) for the assistance I received at that time.

[27]American Nurses' Association Committee on Ethics, 'Statements Regarding Risk vs. Responsibility in Providing Nursing Care', 13 Nov. 1986.

[28]The relevant US regulations are reproduced and discussed in Robert J. Levine, *Ethics and Regulation of Clinical Research* (2nd ed.) (Baltimore: Urban and Schwarzenberg, 1986).

[29]Trevor Hancock, Doug Saunders and Donald Cole, 'Our Chemical Society: Chemicals, Environment and Health', draft report from City of Toronto, Department of Public Health, Health Advocacy Unit, October 1981.

[30]William Lowrance, *Of Acceptable Risk* (Los Altos, CA: Wm. Kaufman Inc., 1976), p. 90.

[31]William Rowe, *An Anatomy of Risk* (New York: John Wiley and Sons, 1977), pp. 52 ff.

[32]Chauncey Starr, 'Benefit-Cost Studies in Sociotechnical Systems', in *Perspectives on Benefit-Risk Decision Making* (Washington, DC: National Academy of Engineering [U.S.], 1972); Paul Slovic, Baruch Fischhoff, and Sarah Lichtenstein, 'Facts and Fears: Understanding Perceived Risk', in R.G. Schwing and W.A. Albers, Jr, eds, *Societal Risk Assessment: How Safe is Safe Enough?* (New York: Plenum Press, 1980).

[33]Mark Sagoff, 'On Markets for Risk', discussion paper, Centre for Philosophy and Public Policy, University of Maryland, p. 14.

[34]The claim is a structural point about justification, *viz.*: to the extent that a risk is occupational in nature, it is *for that reason* voluntarily undergone. Another way of saying the same thing: among the reasons people have for voluntarily assuming risks (including altruistic sacrifice, thrill-seeking, etc.) is to be found the expectation of reimbursement. To say this is not to say that all jobs, and all forms of occupational risk, are equivalent; nor to say that each form of occupational risk, and of reimbursement, as well as combinations of same, are *a priori* justified on balance. The reason why a risk is undergone is only one element in judging whether it was, on balance, voluntarily assumed; among many other suggested factors have been included the context within which the choice of risk is made, alternative decisions available, and the chooser's information about the risk in question.

[35]David Zimmerman, 'Coercive Wage Offers', *Philosophy and Public Affairs* 10, 2 (1981).

[36]Julie Graham and Don Shakow, 'Hazard Pay for Workers: Risk and Reward', *Environment* 23, 8 (October 1981): 14–20 and 44–5.

HIV TESTING
AND CONFIDENTIALITY

H.A. BASSFORD

THE EXPERIENCE OF TESTING

Unlike most Canadians, I have been tested for HIV infection. At the end of a physical examination, I asked my family physician to authorize the test. He was somewhat taken aback, and explained to me that while there was much concern about AIDS, most members of the population had no good reason to be tested, since most people were not at risk. I told him I realized this, but still wished to be tested. This statement was not sufficient to persuade him. His sense of responsibility, both to his patients and to the public purse, would not allow him to order tests unless he believed there were medically acceptable reasons. With this, I explained my reasons, and he authorized the test.

I suspect that the reader is curious about why I needed to be tested. Normally, testing for disease is done in the presence of physical symptoms. The patient presents with an abnormality (e.g., lumps, shortness of breath, fever), and the physician tests for the presence of conditions that may cause these symptoms. But the curiosity in this case will not be about my physical symptoms. Rather it will be about my *social situation*. Am I gay, bisexual (or involved with someone that is), a hemophiliac, a health-care worker?

Am I applying for a new job, for life insurance, to emigrate to another country? AIDS is a disease with very specific modes of transmission, most commonly involving sexual intercourse, so a natural thought will be about my sexual orientation and habits. Thus the very mention of being tested for HIV infection will occasion speculation about intimate and private personal matters.

I work in a university, which is a more open and tolerant environment than most. But I discovered that mentioning my having been tested carried social costs. At the minimum there were jokes about not coming near me. I encountered a wariness of expression, a stiffness of body when shaking hands or giving a hug, out-of-context speculations about other colleagues' sexual preferences, etc. These were mild reactions, but suggest the discomfort around AIDS, and the tendency to connect it with being gay, which carries with it the homophobic attitudes of our society. Rather than document these attitudes here, I shall take for granted the reader's awareness of them.[1] Everyone is aware of food preparers, flight attendants, or health-care workers (to mention three cases in the recent press) who have lost their jobs in Canada because of being HIV-positive. This has happened even given the epidemiological knowledge that the HIV virus is spread only by contact of the blood with infected semen or blood. To quote from the Surgeon General of the United States,[2]

> Everyday living does not present any risk of infection. You cannot get AIDS from casual social contact. . . . Casual social contact such as shaking hands, hugging, social kissing, crying, coughing or sneezing, will not transmit the AIDS virus. Nor has AIDS been contracted from swimming in pools or bathing in hot tubs or from eating in restaurants (even if a restaurant worker has AIDS or carries the AIDS virus). AIDS is not contracted from sharing bed linens, towels, cups, straws, dishes, or any other eating utensils. You cannot get AIDS from toilets, doorknobs, telephones, office machinery, or household furniture. You cannot get AIDS from body massages, masturbation or any non-sexual contact.

Clearly, knowledge about the spread of AIDS has not made it possible for someone who is HIV-positive to live free from irrational social discrimination, should that knowledge become public. Accordingly, there are good reasons for not wishing to publicize one's seropositive status. And indeed, there are good reasons for not telling people even that one has been tested for the presence of HIV.

Sometimes, however, there are also good reasons for wanting to be tested. Although there is at present no cure for AIDS, there are increasing numbers of drugs and medical regimens (such as AZT) that can be effective in postponing the time between the onset of seropositivity and active AIDS. There are thus more and more reasons of medical management that make knowledge desirable. Furthermore, there is the general question of life planning. One of the characteristics of an autonomous, mature individual is the ability to make and live out a life plan. The presence of severe disease requires the rational person to restructure priorities and goals. This is clearly the case with HIV infection. Finally, there is the question of concern for others. A sexually active person may not want to put partners at risk, or may wish to be sure they are aware of the risk involved. Someone may be contemplating a monogamous relationship, and want to be sure it is safe to stop using the usual protective devices. A couple, or a woman, may want to make sure that there is no risk to a potential child. In all these cases, if there is a risk of infection, then there is reason to find out whether such infection is present. The question for the person who wishes a test is how to gain the knowledge without encountering the very real social problems I have delineated above.

PHYSICIAN CONFIDENTIALITY

While it is perhaps possible to avoid this stigma in everyday life by simply not telling people about being tested, it is not easy to maintain such privacy in the confines of the doctor's office. It is important to see that this is not because of any prurient interest on the physician's part, but rather is required in order to provide proper health care. The social function of the medical profession is to maintain or restore the health of individuals, and as far as possible to alleviate illness-based suffering. For them to get the information they need, they have to examine us physically, often in ways that would not be allowed to others. They sometimes have to be told of our emotional pressures and of our personal lifestyles, how we eat, how we exercise, how we perform personal hygiene, and even what our sexual practices are. Thus in order to do their job, doctors must often be given very personal information.

What of my own request for an HIV test? My physician realized that the very fact of requesting such a test showed that I was concerned about the possibility of having contracted AIDS. He also realized that there was tremendous general fear about this disease, with many people having quite irrational personal fears. Was I in this position? If so, what I needed was information and counselling rather than, or at least prior to, testing. On the other hand, I might be at risk, in which case he would want to talk to me about the degree of risk, to prepare and support me psychologically around the testing, and perhaps to counsel me as to how to protect myself and others. His ability to carry out his caring function is thus dependent upon his gathering specific and possibly intimate information from me.

I gave information to my physician, as patients generally do to their physicians, because I trusted his judgement that he needed this information in order to provide proper health care. I also trusted that he would not use this information to my detriment. The personal and private knowledge that doctors gain from their patients allows them to provide treatment but also gives them tremendous power over those patients. Indeed, their power goes

beyond that of information. Patients often come to physicians in very vulnerable states. They are ill, not able to exercise their normal control over their
lives, and so more than usually vulnerable. They are examined in a gown, in
the physician's office or in hospital, in trappings and situations wherein they
do not feel themselves to be in charge. They are medically untrained, and
must rely upon the physician's expertise. Both literally and figuratively,
patients must place themselves in their doctors' hands.

Because of all this, the physician has a strong moral obligation to confidentiality. The doctor's professional commitment to patient care can be accomplished only if the patient gives information freely, and this will be best
accomplished if it is clear that such information will be held in confidence.
Moreover, the human situation of the doctor-patient relationship requires
confidentiality. Doctors accept patients, with all their vulnerabilities, into
their care; patients entrust themselves to their physicians. Should doctors
take advantage of patients' vulnerabilities, they are violating the trust that
they have accepted both in undertaking to treat a particular patient and in
entering a profession that essentially involves such relationships. Physicians
take immoral advantage of their power relationships if they have sexual
relations with their patients. They also do so if they do not respect the privacy
of information provided in the examining room. It can accordingly be seen
that the doctor-patient relationship is a fiduciary one, with the proper practice of medicine depending upon the doctor's being trustworthy, holding
information in strict confidence, and not taking advantage of the patient's
vulnerability. From the Hippocratic Oath onward, medical codes of ethics
have emphasized this, medical associations have attempted to enforce it, and
medical schools have inculcated it.

What does this mean with respect to HIV testing? The goal of the patient is
to receive relevant information and care without encountering the discriminatory social practices that unfortunately now exist. The Canadian AIDS
Society has proposed that this is best accomplished by instituting a testing
procedure for the AIDS antibody 'that is completely anonymous'.[3] Some such
clinics have been set up in Canada; many exist in the United States. Individuals are allowed to give a pseudonym or number, and though they may receive
pre- or post-test counselling, they do so without anyone's knowing their
identity. This option allows individuals to control personal information and
thus avoid social discrimination. Given that many people at risk for HIV
infection are members of groups that have been constantly subject to discrimination and prejudice, it is a good idea *not* to require them to be dependent upon a physician's good will. Thus there should be anonymous testing
available.

But such complete anonymity is not the best solution for most people.
With the growing numbers of research results, there is good reason to maintain medical monitoring of HIV infection, in order for individuals to have
access both to developing information and to developing treatment. This is

very difficult in the absence of any case records or of access to the patient by the treating physician. The best way to effect this is to re-emphasize, in the case of HIV testing and monitoring, the tradition of physician confidentiality, and see to it that, to quote the Canadian AIDS Society's second preference, 'the client's identity is known only to the testing physician'. This would involve maintaining much of the process of anonymous testing. The physician must take care to keep confidential information from office staff. Technicians do not have reasons to know the identities of people being tested, so anonymity should be maintained during visits to laboratories and on papers sent to such institutions. But given this change in process, this proposal would both work in the patient's interest and help to maintain the traditionally significant ethical doctor-patient relationship.

Unfortunately, this ideal does not now exist. Principle six of the Canadian Medical Association Code of Ethics reads, 'An ethical physician will keep in confidence information derived from his [*sic*] patient, or from a colleague, regarding a patient and divulge it only with the permission of the patient except when the law requires him to do so.' In all ten provinces AIDS is a reportable disease, which means that the physician is legally required to report AIDS-related patient information, usually including the patient's identity, to the medical health officer. In six provinces HIV seropositivity is also reportable.[4] This means that the CMA partially exempts physicians from patient confidentiality in the case of AIDS and HIV seropositivity, extending the range of knowledge to another set of individuals.

This extension takes place because AIDS is a communicable disease, and as such is considered a danger to the public health; hence it falls within the purview of those whose job it is to protect the health of the public. In the case of communicable diseases, various means have traditionally been taken to effect public protection, including the collection of epidemiological data, education in prevention, voluntary or involuntary treatment or immunization, voluntary or involuntary screening, contact tracing, and quarantine of individuals or groups. Two problems accordingly arise for the person undergoing HIV testing. Will the public health system keep the desired confidences? Will that system itself subject patients to unwarranted coercion or invasions of privacy? I shall address these questions by first considering the moral propriety of the greatest interventions, involuntary mass-screening and quarantine, and then proceeding to examine the lesser interventions into patient privacy.

QUARANTINE

The most invasive response to AIDS has been that of Cuba, which has instituted the world's only nation-wide compulsory testing program. Those who test positive are subjected to lifetime quarantine in designated areas, where they are well-fed and well-housed, receive excellent medical care, and are allowed visits from family and friends. The quarantine is thus as humane as it is possible for any quarantine to be.[5] Nonetheless, the fact remains that those quarantined are being denied significant personal freedoms, based upon the need to protect the public from harm. Is this justified? I shall argue that it is not.

I propose two principles. The first I shall term the 'foundational principle'. The moral purpose of civil society is to allow people to live well: to have their physical necessities met, to develop their human potential, to share in the joys of community. Such a society works best when founded upon a principle of mutual trust and respect, with the rights to privacy, self-determination, and freedom being overridable only when other people's rights are deliberately or negligently infringed or when their safety is clearly threatened. Reflection will show that both criminal and tort law are based upon this principle. While the state can legitimately interfere with the behaviour of adults, it must shoulder the burden of proof by showing that one of the above conditions applies. In modern societies rights are adopted not out of a desire to let people selfishly pursue their own interests, but rather out of a respect for people and a belief that they for the most part will handle their own affairs decently.

The second principle is as follows: when it is necessary to interfere with liberty, such interference should use the least restrictive alternative.[6] The point of this principle is straightforward. When there are two competing values, then even though one supersedes the other, there are cases wherein aspects of the other can be retained, and if possible they should be. To take an example from the current discussion, if public safety from a disease can be achieved by identifying and educating those spreading the disease rather than by identifying and quarantining them, then the proper path is to educate them.

With these principles in mind, let me now look at quarantine and universal mandatory testing. Is the public at risk of significant harm from those seropositive for HIV? It is clearly not at risk because of their mere physical presence in society. This could be the case with a virulent air-borne plague, with which people could become infected by merely being in the same space as those already infected. This might have been the case for Mary Mallon (Typhoid Mary), who was quarantined in 1915 for the involuntary spread of typhoid fever. In such cases quarantine might be justified, even though those spreading the disease intend no harm whatsoever. However, the contagiousness of HIV is a very different matter. As my earlier reference to the Surgeon General of the United States has shown, AIDS is not spread by normal social contact. It is spread *only* through anal or vaginal sexual intercourse, or through the intermingling of blood through sharing intravenous needles, blood transfusions, or major health-care accidents. People who have been found HIV-positive can produce infection, and thus cause harm, only by these means. Thus they can have their rights overridden only if they are engaging in these sorts of activities in ways which recklessly or purposely put others at risk.

But quarantine upon evidence of seropositivity presumes that all such individuals will in fact deliberately or negligently spread the disease. It presumes that everyone who is HIV-positive is of immoral and vicious character. Such a presumption is itself morally odious. It goes beyond even the prejudice that people with AIDS 'deserve what they get' because they have engaged in 'immoral' behaviour, and like this prejudice is reflective of the hysteria and homophobia that all too often have surfaced with respect to AIDS. It is also clearly factually false. Public health officers universally submit that the number of people with AIDS who want to spread the disease is extremely small.[7] Jeff Levi of the National Gay Task Force has put the reason clearly: 'No one knows better than [those with AIDS] how terrible the disease is, and they wouldn't want to spread it.'[8] To stigmatize people who are HIV-positive, and to quarantine them on unfounded presumptions of moral odiousness, flies in the face of the foundational principle of human society, and is accordingly not a morally acceptable practice.

This argument militates as well against preventive quarantine of any targeted high-risk group. Hemophiliacs, gays, or intravenous drug users (commonly mentioned as high-risk) are all groups made up of extremely varied individuals. Although some members of those groups may act viciously or recklessly, the great majority will not do so. Accordingly, even if such groups could be identified for mandatory testing (which would be very nearly impossible at best, and which would require massive state intervention into private behaviour), preventive quarantine of HIV-positive members of these groups would be morally wrong. Prediction of dangerousness has been found by the criminal justice system to be notoriously difficult, which is why preventive punishment has been rejected and only those found guilty of actually committing crimes have their liberty restricted. Such should be the case in the prevention of the spread of AIDS.

There are also empirical considerations concerning the testing procedures that militate against both universal testing and quarantine. The ELISA test, which is the most widely used, meets most epidemiological screening standards. However, for formal statistical reasons, its predictive value (the probability that a property is in fact present given a positive test result) decreases when the test is applied to the general population, in which the frequency of HIV infection is overall quite low.[9] In testing the general population of Canada, one-half to two-thirds of the positive results will be false positive. That is, more than one-half of the individuals who get a positive result will be virus-free. Retesting, or testing with one of the other available tests as well, will very significantly reduce the number of false positives, but the fact remains that the predictive value will never reach 100 per cent. Reasonable numbers of false positives are acceptable in some cases. When the Red Cross screens all donated blood, the presence of numbers of false positives means they will not use some blood that is safe to use. This loss is acceptable, given that sufficient blood is available and that they want to be very sure of screening out blood that is HIV-infected. However, if coercive measures are taken, based upon test results, then significant numbers of people (especially when it is considered that entire populations are being tested) will be severely restricted, even though they cannot put anyone at risk. This result is not acceptable.

MANDATORY SCREENING

Moreover, given the moral non-viability of quarantine, there is little point to large-scale mandatory screening. What will it mean for the public health goal of halting the spread of the disease when people are identified as carrying AIDS antibodies? They can't be treated, for there is no treatment; they can't be quarantined or otherwise stigmatized, for this is immoral. What is left is the gathering of data for epidemiological study, contact tracing in order to warn others, and counselling those found to be seropositive so they will not spread the condition. I shall argue that the costs, both social and economic, are too high, given the possible results. Further, the same goals can be achieved just as well by less intrusive means, and so, by the principle of the least restrictive alternative, these are the means that should be used.

Let me look first at the costs. Testing the entire population would cost well over a hundred million dollars, purely in laboratory fees. It would require a massive increase in laboratory facilities, and a major bureaucracy and policing mechanism to see to it that the population complied with the testing requirement. This would not be cheap, either in dollars or in social costs. The entire population would go through the anxiety of waiting for results. Over half of those initially testing positive would be false positive; they and their relations would undergo immense stress while waiting retesting. Given that most people are not greatly at risk, and that risk can be very significantly reduced by voluntary changes in personal behaviour (safe sex, not sharing needles), one wonders if such stresses are justified.

The spectre of unnecessary suffering for the seropositive also arises once more. The largest seropositive group in Canada is composed of gay men, who as such have been historically subjected to much social and legal discrimination. They and others would legitimately fear that surveillance could easily turn to more restrictive actions. Additionally, it is hard to imagine that the public's already existing prejudice and fear would not increase if the government implemented a massive program based upon a perceived need to track down all possible sources of infection. Further, the mechanism required to complete the screening, given the numbers of people involved, and the size of the resulting government data bank, full of highly personal information, would make it extremely difficult, if not impossible, to maintain confidentiality. This would increase the already existing discriminatory practices with respect to employment, service delivery, housing, etc. Taken together, these are very high moral costs.

But additionally there is the problem of whether the program could achieve its goals. People who fear or otherwise strongly oppose a program can hardly be expected to co-operate wholeheartedly with it. Some would try to evade the program completely; others would not volunteer information, or would deliberately misinform (e.g., officials will not know our sex partners unless we identify them); the co-operation necessary for successful counselling or education would not likely be forthcoming. Yet such co-operation is crucial if the program is to succeed. The point has been well put by David J. Mayo:[10]

> Since no vaccine or cure for AIDS is available, the most promising strategy available for cutting down on the transmission of AIDS now is the reduction of high-risk activities, and this can be achieved only through cooperation and education of high-risk groups about what activities are unsafe. This task is already well underway in the gay community in some cities, but is obviously frustrated by any antagonism between public officials and high-risk groups. Mutual trust is absolutely essential if individuals are to begin to listen to, believe, and finally act on the advice of health professionals about what activities are unsafe. That is virtually impossible when those at risk are – or believe they are – stigmatized as 'outsiders'. That is the nearly unanimous belief of those who actually work in public health with victims of stigmatizing diseases, particularly diseases associated with stigmatized behaviour.

From all this it appears that the results of required screening contradict the goals of such screening. When the moral improprieties of mandatory testing are added, it becomes clear that alternative policies should be investigated.

EDUCATION AND SOCIAL SUPPORT

What is required is a policy that combines voluntary, truly confidential testing, comprehensive education, and some supportive social programs. The primary goal, to reduce the spread of AIDS, can be accomplished if those who engage in potentially infective activities, whether HIV-positive or -negative, modify their behaviour patterns. There is clear evidence that carefully constructed educational programs can lead to safer sexual behaviour.[11] Especially effective are those programs conducted by, or in combination with, relevant community organizations. To quote from Ronald Bayer:

> it was stunning to find that in the face of the AIDS epidemic volunteer efforts undertaken by community organizations and funded in the most limited way by public agencies had apparently produced dramatic, even unprecedented changes in the sexual behaviour of gay men.[12]

Peer-group and other innovative educational techniques can help people to gain the knowledge and motivation to reassess the meaning of their behaviour, to act both in their own interest and out of concern for others. It must not be thought this is an easy process. Many men, surely including some readers of this paper, refuse to wear condoms. This is to refuse to accept responsibility for the results of their sexuality. Many women are socialized or coerced into compliance. Accordingly, successful educational programs to combat AIDS must do more than provide information; they must actively face deep-seated questions of gender and heterosexual sexual politics. Such programs may be expensive, although cheaper than quarantine and universal testing; but morally they are much preferable to the alternatives, not least because they address long-standing social injustices. When access to the physical means to change behaviour, such as needle-exchange programs and the placing of condom-vending machines in high-school washrooms, is combined with such educational programs, there can be significant progress towards slowing the spread of AIDS.

The notion of trust and co-operation should be emphasized here. The most successful programs are those wherein the government and the affected communities work together. In such cases those groups affected or most at risk can readily perceive that the authorities act out of concern for them, and do so in a context of respecting their personhood and sense of personal responsibility. This is also true with voluntary testing. The voluntary patient is more likely to work with the physician, and so to benefit from the physician's counselling or from the counselling arranged by the physician with relevant peer groups.

The opposite is the case with required testing. The coerced person will be seen as untrustworthy or unable to act autonomously. Being so seen does not tend to make one co-operative, nor does it engender the confidence and self-respect needed to cope with the situation. A voluntary testing program is consistent with the 'foundation principle'; an involuntary one is not. Moreover, the results of voluntary testing, when combined with education, are at least as good. The conclusion is that voluntary testing with maintenance of primary physician confidentiality is the preferred social policy.

However, it might be argued that this conclusion is too strong. While the proposed program provides for better behaviour modification, it does not provide for proper collection of epidemiological data or for the contact tracing necessary to protect others. Because of this, some sort of mandatory testing, or at least required reporting to public health authorities of positive results, is necessary.

These considerations are not decisive. Epidemiological data are often essential to understanding and conquering a disease. It is important to know the ways in which the disease is spread and the ways in which individual instances of the disease develop. But the gathering of this information does not require officers of public health to know the identities of those whose cases provide data. The Centres for Disease Control in the United States, for example, have devised a reporting mechanism that allows reporting without the use of names or other personal identifiers, but that precludes duplicate reporting. Even though this method is more complex, it neither interferes with privacy nor produces non-compliance and false reporting, and so it is the morally proper choice.

This is also the case with contact tracing. The closest parallel is the use of contact tracing for venereal diseases, which has long been a standard practice. It has not, however, always been clearly successful, as Allan Brandt reports in his history of venereal disease in the United States:[13]

> The ultimate effect of case-finding remains difficult to evaluate. . . . Contact epidemiology clearly brought many unsuspecting individuals into treatment before they could spread their infections to others. But the knowledge that information regarding contacts would be sought by public health professionals also had the effect of encouraging some individuals to seek the aid of quacks or private practitioners who guaranteed absolute confidentiality. Indeed, most private physicians have resisted public health requirements that they report individuals suffering from venereal disease to public officials so that contacts can be approached.

While contact tracing did alert many, it drove others away from the health-care and education system. The Surgeon General of the United States believes that this can also happen with contact tracing for those who are HIV-positive, and for this reason opposes reporting to and tracing by public health departments.[14] It also can drive people away in another sense. Since affected communities are strongly opposed to this requirement, its imposition would not further the crucially needed community co-operation in education and counselling. As a social policy, public health contact tracing might well carry more costs than it produces benefits.

Moreover, a reasonable voluntary alternative exists. For the most part, officials will be able to find out who our sexual contacts are only if we tell them. Public health officers will be able to carry out their goal of contact tracing only if HIV-positive individuals volunteer the relevant information. In a coercive situation, fearing that friends and lovers will be 'listed' or have their privacy dangerously invaded (think of a lover with a sensitive job), many will not volunteer accurate information. On the other hand, as I have emphasized often in this essay, most people do not want to cause harm to others. With appropriate counselling and support, it is reasonable to think that most will be willing to inform their sexual partners, even though this will sometimes be difficult for them. In some cases, people may find they need the help of their physician or a specially trained person in informing partners. This kind of help can be provided without keeping lists and with minimum loss of confidentiality.

While this voluntary method of contact tracing would not mean that all those at risk of infection would be informed, it should be as successful as the mandatory contact-tracing method. On the one hand, the mandatory method would inform, as the voluntary method would not, sexual partners of those who could not be persuaded to inform their partners themselves, but who could be coerced into giving their names. On the other hand, the mandatory method would not reach the sexual partners of those who would stay away from the system or would withhold information. The mandatory method also alienates communities with whom co-operation is important. Given all this, and given that the voluntary system is far less invasive of privacy than the mandatory one, the principle of the least restrictive alternative prescribes opting for the voluntary system. With this result, the overall conclusion can now be stated. The best social policy for HIV-testing is one that makes testing voluntary, that maintains physician-patient confidentiality, and that does not involve mandatory reporting to or contact tracing by officers of public health.

THE PHYSICIAN'S DUTY TO WARN

In closing, I wish to look at a widely debated situation, that of the 'noncompliant positive'. There are some people who, knowing they are HIV-positive, will continue to engage in high-risk sexual activities, without informing their partners of the risk. They will, that is, do what I have consistently argued that the vast majority of people will not do; they will deliberately or recklessly endanger others. Such cases catch the public's attention, and much debate is focused upon them. It is easy to see why: everyone feels threatened. But it must be kept in mind that very few of us are actually so threatened. As was earlier pointed out, public health officials consider such cases very rare. Not many people want to inflict such suffering on others. By far the greater threat comes from having unprotected sex with people who do not know that they are infected. This is risked every time we have intercourse without a condom.

People who know they are HIV-positive and endanger others are acting immorally, and indeed numbers of them have quite properly been charged under the Criminal Code.[15] But the public must not think that dealing with this small group will resolve the problem. If we do not know our HIV status and have unprotected sex, then *we* are acting immorally. Every time a man refuses to wear a condom, he is acting immorally. Educational programs and social dialogue should constantly bring this fact home. The realities of AIDS, that is, can be addressed only by a social reassessment of our sexual politics.

With this background, I now turn to a much discussed version of this case wherein the principle of physician confidentiality can, I think, sometimes be overridden. Consider the following scenario. A patient comes for testing, and is found to be seropositive. During counselling it becomes clear that the patient has a partner who believes the patient is monogamous, and that in this belief the two regularly engage in unprotected sex. The patient *insists* that the partner not be warned. What is the physician to do?

Normally, we all have a duty to warn those who are unknowingly at risk. We yell out to warn a person who doesn't see a car bearing down on them. If someone drunkenly announces he is going over to 'punch out' an acquaintance, we telephone the acquaintance. If we do not do so, we know that we must shoulder moral blame apart from that carried by the person committing the harm. Because of our knowledge and inaction, we morally become part of the causal chain leading to harm.

Physicians, like everyone else, have a duty to warn. The question is, however, what the moral weighting is when the duty to warn conflicts with the physician's duty of confidentiality to a patient. The duty to confidentiality is very strong, but not morally absolute. As seen earlier in the paper, it arises out of the conditions necessary for treatment and a respect for the vulnerability and autonomy of the patient. But concern for treating a patient is not more important than protecting innocent people from extreme harm, and in those very rare cases wherein preserving confidentiality will clearly lead to such harm, the confidentiality must yield. If a psychiatrist's patient explains just how he or she has committed a series of unsolved killings, then talks of the next victim, the psychiatrist must act to protect the victim, even if this sets back or makes impossible the patient's ongoing treatment.

The problem lies in deciding when such a case exists. In the above example the answer is clear. It would also be clear if the patient were relating dreams of violence that in the psychiatrist's judgement were not serious threats. But in between lies a considerable grey area, wherein the physician must make difficult case-by-case judgements of the probability and degree of harm. These situations will be ones for individual moral judgement rather than general social policy.

This will be so with most questions of whether to warn the sexual partner of HIV-positive patients who are unwilling to reveal their status to the partner. The sexual partner is running a risk, the results of which can be very grave, but the case is not immediately comparable to the one of homicide, above. First, HIV seropositivity is not an automatic sentence of death, since only one out of three who are seropositive develops AIDS within seven years.[16] Second, each sexual act carries a fairly small probability of infection. Third, the partner may already be seropositive. These considerations do not mean there is not sufficient dangerousness to require a warning, but they do mean that the physician can take time to think out the proper intervention.

Several questions can be investigated. What is the source of the patient's reluctance? Will counselling overcome it? Is there a way to reveal the risk to the partner without the results the patient fears? Can the patient find a way to modify sex practices, or temporarily refrain from sex, while this matter is being worked out? In short, education and counselling should not be immediately abandoned. The patient can be given time to get used to the situation, and to be persuaded that the physician will be a support during the ongoing difficulties. The physician has time to use the authority conferred by the doctor–patient relationship to produce the morally best result.

It may become clear that the patient is emotionally unable to disclose or to authorize disclosure, or, indeed, is simply bad-willed. In such cases, if the physician has been able to judge that the partner is involuntarily at risk, then a warning will become morally appropriate. But even when the duty of confidentiality is overridden by the duty to warn, this should be done in such a way as to maximize the possibility of patient care. If the patient is told of the physician's decision (and so can prepare for what is coming), is invited to take part, and is provided with assurances of psycho-social backup, then many of the concerns upon which the duty of physician confidentiality is based can still be met, and the minimum moral damage caused to occur in what will necessarily be a very unhappy situation.

It might be argued that under these conditions of confidentiality some people will refuse to be tested, and that people who know they are seropositive always have the possibility of warning their partners, whereas untested people do not.[17] This may well be true, but it is not persuasive, given the overall proposals of the paper. First, as independently argued earlier, there should be clinics that provide anonymous testing. People who fear that this very specific exception to confidentiality will affect them will have access to the clinics and will be in the position outlined above. Second, many of the people who pose the present dilemma for physicians are in some sense asking for help. If they were not, they could pretty simply lie – could say they had told their partners, were refraining from sex, only had safe sex, etc. – and the dilemma would not arise. Most of those wanting help, even if this desire were not fully conscious, would still come to a general practitioner. Given these considerations, it can be concluded that the above argument does not justify a requirement of confidentiality such that some doctors must live with the terrible moral burden of knowing that they were in a position to have warned specific, clearly threatened, innocent individuals about grievous harm, but because they were doctors did not do so.

I shall close with one general observation. The awful dilemmas just discussed, as well as many others around AIDS, often arise because of fears of having sexual practices and preferences revealed. Such fears are usually well founded, arising from the prejudices and intolerance of our society. AIDS is a terrible medical tragedy, but it focuses our attention upon a terrible social tragedy as well. So, while we can often sort out the morally least damaging path through the particular dilemmas of AIDS treatment, our goal should always be to change those social attitudes and conditions that cause them to arise.

NOTES

[1]For an excellent study of AIDS and homophobia, see Dennis Altman, *AIDS and the New Puritanism* (London: Pluto Press, 1986).

[2]*Surgeon General's Report on Acquired Immune Deficiency Syndrome* (Washington, DC: United States Government), p. 21.

[3]Canadian AIDS Society, 'Guidelines on Voluntary HIV Antibody Testing', January 1988.

[4]D.G. Casswell, 'Disclosure by a Physician of AIDS-Related Patient Information: An Ethical and Legal Dilemma', *The Canadian Bar Review* 68, 2 (June 1989): 256-7.

[5]Even though I shall be extremely critical of the quarantine program, it must be emphasized that this does not constitute an overall condemnation of Cuba's AIDS program. Cubans with AIDS all receive high-quality medical care, which cannot be said of any other Third World country. Indeed, the United States does not compare all that well in this particular. Given the user-pay medical system, the fact that many people with AIDS live in big-city ghettos, and that many others exhaust their resources long before they no longer need medical care, many Americans with AIDS cannot be said to receive high-quality medical care.

[6]This is a more general version of a principle proposed for public health restrictions in Lawrence O. Gostin, William J. Curran, and Mary E. Clark, 'The Case Against Compulsory Casefinding in Controlling AIDS – Testing, Screening and Reporting', *American Journal of Law & Medicine* 12, 1: 24.

[7]Ronald Bayer, *Private Acts, Social Consequences: AIDS and the Politics of Public Health* (New York: Free Press, 1989), pp. 156, 192, 198.

[8]Ibid., p. 193.

[9]The explanation of the relevant statistical concepts most accessible to the layperson can be found in Kenneth R. Howe, 'Why Mandatory Screening for AIDS is a Very Bad Idea', in Christine Pierce and Donald VanDeVeer, *AIDS: Ethics and Public Policy* (Belmont, CA: Wadsworth, 1988), pp. 140-9.

[10]David J. Mayo, 'AIDS, Quarantines, and Noncompliant Positives', in Pierce and VanDeVeer, pp. 117-18.

[11]See, for example, Ronald O. Valdiserri, *et al.*, 'AIDS Prevention in Homosexual and Bisexual Men: Results of Randomized Trial Evaluating Two Risk Reduction Interventions', *AIDS* 3, 1 (Jan. 1989): 21-6.

[12]Bayer, p. 226. See also Altman, Ch. 5.

[13]Allan M. Brandt, *No Magic Bullet: A Social History of Venereal Disease in the United States Since 1880* (New York: Oxford University Press, 1987), p. 151.

[14]*Surgeon General's Report*, p. 30.

[15]It might be argued that these cases, when discovered, should be dealt with by means of quarantine. While I do not have space to argue the case properly here, I agree with Wendy Parmet that the criminal law has moral advantages here. As she

says, 'The criminal law would punish only those individuals who were found after a full trial to have committed clearly proscribed acts. A criminal statute would not rely, as might a quarantine, on uncertain predictions of future behavior and less than full procedural protections' ('AIDS and Quarantine: The Revival of an Archaic Doctrine', *Hofstra Law Review* [Fall 1985]: 85–6).

[16] Royal Society of Canada, *AIDS: A Perspective for Canadians (Summary Report and Recommendations)* (Ottawa 1988), p. 3.

[17] Casswell, p. 248.

CATASTROPHIC RIGHTS: VITAL PUBLIC INTERESTS AND CIVIL LIBERTIES IN CONFLICT

JOHN DIXON

CHEATERS AND REBELS

The ethical questions associated with the issue of freedom of access to experimental drugs were dramatically, albeit unintentionally, posed by an edition of DIMENSIONS, the special newspaper of the Fifth International Conference on AIDS in Montreal. The 7 June 1989 issue of the paper carried a story reporting the findings of Dr Margaret Fischl, of the University of Miami School of Medicine, concerning the importance of early treatment of AIDS with the drug AZT.[1] Fischl found that the greatest impact of AZT occurs during the first six to eighteen months of treatment, and the greatest effect is on patients with the first signs of AIDS symptoms. The same article reported the findings of Dr Douglas Richman and his co-workers at the University of California, who found a tenfold increase in resistance to AZT in patients who had received the drug for six to twelve months. The clear implication of this article was that, in HIV infection, the earliest possible intervention with anti-virals was a logically compelling option to explore.

But if persons living with AIDS (PLWAs) at the conference took the findings of Fischl and Richman 'personally' – that is, as information important to their individual choices as they sought treatment – *DIMENSIONS* had a front-page story on the same day that struck a discordant note.

The article began: 'Dr Ian Weller warned at Tuesday's plenary session that the use of investigational drugs as conventional treatment and the practice of preventative treatment in asymptomatic individuals was making it increasingly difficult to judge accurately the efficacy of new drugs.'[2] Dr Weller, from the Middlesex School of Medicine in the UK, emphasized that 'he was not speaking only for himself, but was presenting a consensus opinion derived from consultations taken over the last months with colleagues in several countries'.[3] All of these scientists were worried about the emergence of a research environment that was becoming patient–driven rather than effectively controlled by the scientific and political elements of our therapeutic system. AIDS drugs were threatening to become ungovernable.

What was happening was precisely what one would expect rational PLWAs to do in the face of even the rumour of findings such as were formally reported by Fischl and Richman at the conference. Realizing that anti-virals may offer a limited window of opportunity through which to attack AIDS before the disease developed a resistance to the treatment, both the sick and the 'worried well' were trying to beat their deadly foe to the punch.

Many of the PLWAs at the Montreal conference wore 'SILENCE = DEATH' lapel buttons, and they were speedily feeding news of the latest findings into their international network of patient coalitions and 'buyers clubs'. More HIV-infected individuals would soon be practising 'preventive treatment' in an effort to save their lives, thus disqualifying themselves as subjects for any controlled and blinded experiments of these new therapeutic options. What is potentially worse, subjects in ongoing trials would be more likely to 'cheat' – i.e., to take extra or unapproved drugs without telling the investigators – and thus compromise the experiment. This has already become a bigger problem with subjects in trials of AIDS drugs than medical scientists have ever experienced with any other group.

This is a serious matter, since medical progress on HIV infection is directly dependent upon the ability of medical researchers to conduct experiments that are genuinely scientific. The 'gold standard' of methodology in drug research, Dr Robert Levine of Yale forcefully emphasized at the Montreal conference, is the double-blinded, randomized experiment.[4] In its classic simplicity, this involves the inclusion of only those subjects who satisfy a carefully predetermined standard of relevant homogeneity – i.e., all with about the same stage of disease development, same history of treatment or non-treatment, etc. – and then their separation into two distinct arms. One group of subjects receives the experimental drug, and is called the experimental arm. The other group of subjects receives the control substance (either a placebo or the established therapy), and is called the control arm. The selection of subjects for the different arms is made as perfectly random as possible in order to control such possible human variables as, say, an investigator's unconsciously placing the most likeable subjects in the experimental arm. And the experiment is double-blinded in that it is arranged so that neither the investigators nor the subjects know who is in which arm, thus controlling the range of human variables associated with expectation and hope in both groups.

The 'gold standard' trial guards, most obviously, against the well-understood placebo effect. However, the case for experimental controls is further strengthened when one recognizes that a significant improvement in treatment might still be small enough to escape detection against the background of an imperfect grasp of the natural history of a disease. This was the point emphasized by Dr Weller in Montreal when he complained of the increasing difficulty involved for investigators who must be alert not simply to some gross result such as whether the subject is completely cured, but also to the appearance of conditions that may only indirectly suggest an improvement ('surrogate markers', in the jargon). Such subtle effects of treatment might, of course, escape investigators even in a controlled setting; but the best chance of catching a slight but significant effect (which could lead to other hypotheses and experiments that build on that knowledge) is in the most carefully controlled setting possible.

Subject discipline is a vital consideration in such experimentation. If subjects discover which arm they are in, or take drugs other than those prescribed by the experimental design, the results can be compromised (i.e., there may be effects observed that are attributable not to the experimental drug, but to uncontrolled variables), and at least a portion of the scientific objective lost. In a demanding research environment, that portion may be all the advantage that science can give us, and losing it can amount to losing our ability to make medical progress. It was this consideration that prompted Yale's Levine to argue at Montreal that the oft-posed conflict between ethical principles and strictly controlled human experimentation was really a pseudo-conflict, since controls are an indispensable element of our ability to gain a public health benefit – medical mastery of catastrophic illnesses. (An illness is catastrophic in direct proportion to the emergent threat it poses to the life expectancy of a particular patient. Although I will not pause to discuss it here, this depends upon several factors – most obviously, the natural history of the fatal illness, the age and general health of the patient, and the state of the relevant medical arts. A middle-aged person with his or her first opportunistic AIDS-related illness is, in 1990, definitive of my conception of catastrophic illness.) Compromising our ability to effectively seek the goal of medical mastery could mean the practical loss of any realistic prospect of safe and effective treatment for AIDS, a disease that can be counted upon to cause incalculable human suffering. Permitting that to happen was, Levine insisted, unethical.

Against this logic, some PLWAs and their advocates responded that the heart of the matter for them was not the necessity of controlled experimentation, or even the use of placebo controls where there is no established therapy, but the issue of *coerced* participation in the trial of catastrophic drugs.[5] To the claim of researchers that they experimented only on volunteers, and that 'nobody put a gun to their heads', PLWAs countered that it was their catastrophic prognosis that put them under the gun. It was AIDS itself that turned the conditions of randomization and blindness into a 'godfather offer' that simply couldn't be refused, because refusal meant – for them, at least – the death of hope that is associated with a new drug. Hence, as they would have it, they enter into the same kind of 'voluntary' undertakings as do the starving poor of Calcutta, who seek the opportunity to sell enough of their blood to ensure both the temporary survival of their families and their own probable death. Nobody has to coerce them; they bring their own vulnerability to be taken advantage of. In the face of such circumstantial coercion we should, they contend, speak not of 'cheaters' but of 'rebels'.

There was also, as I argued at the Montreal conference, something missing in Levine's argument: due notice of the difference between the *interests* of PLWAs in therapeutic autonomy, as distinct from their *rights* to such freedom. Of this claim, more in a moment. First, though, it is important to recognize that the regulation of experimental drugs is a long-standing governmental practice, legitimized by a wide range of public-interest considerations. Any newly minted right in this area must confront a well-established public health currency. So a brief digression is in order, to sympathetically place Levine's argument in its appropriate general context, and to prepare the ground for the introduction of the special ethical considerations associated with catastrophic illness.

ONCE BURNED ... THE CASE FOR REGULATORY CONSERVATISM

There are at least three overlapping categories of public health interests associated with the regulation of drugs: the protection of people, the conservation of health-care resources, and the maintenance of our ability to do science.

The protection of people. Just as we do not have to take complete individual responsibility for determining the quality and wholesomeness of the canned tuna we buy at the corner store, we can expect that the drugs sold by our pharmacist have been judged safe and effective by the federal government. We take this for granted until we travel to other jurisdictions in which a visit to the drug store can be a many-splendoured and dangerous consumer outing – giving fresh meaning to the invitation to 'shop till you drop'. The provision of such regulatory protection is at least colourable as paternalism, a limitation of the freedom of persons 'for their own good'. However, and to the extent that it is actually paternalistic, the regulation of the sale of drugs provides an enormous measure of safety and convenience to the citizenry. We may rouse our absolutist democratic sensibilities when considering a limitation upon *fundamental* freedoms, such as freedom of conscience and expression; but we have traditionally permitted a narrow range of governmental paternalism when the demonstrable public benefits gained by it are both substantial and historically established.

The protection of our limited health-care resources. The power of our therapeutic system is intimately linked with the power of our medicines. To the extent that we have and use safe and effective drugs to treat the sick, there is proportionally less consumption of our limited ability to palliate and maintain them. And to the extent that we have and use safe and effective palliative and maintaining treatments when, as is too often true, we cannot cure, we have more resources left to use in those most demanding cases for which we have no such medicines. Directly or indirectly, we all must pay for the therapeutic misadventures of those who gamble on unapproved treatments and fail. This is not a consideration restricted to churlish hearts, but a definite limiting factor in the ability of any present society to care for the health of its members. Seen in this light, the regulation of drugs is an essential feature of a responsible governance of our general ability, as a society, to discharge our health-care obligations.

The protection of our ability to do science. I have already touched on this above. This seemingly abstract notion has enormous practical importance in connection with questions of public health interests versus individual freedom because, as we have seen, the *scientific* determination of the safety and efficacy of experimental drugs depends upon carefully controlled study. If we are to have medical progress, we must have science; and if we are to have science, we must have experimental controls. Unhappily, the antiseptic notion of the control of studies rather quickly translates into the troubling reality of the control of persons.

As a *general* consideration, however, this instance of society getting organized around a communal purpose is clearly just another good idea at work rather than a dramatic slice of 'civilization and its discontents'. Consider, for instance, the people who suffer from migraine headaches (as many as 15 per cent of North Americans). Each of these individual sufferers has a pressing individual interest in obtaining fast relief, and each will certainly be inclined to try different therapies in an effort to find something that works. If we leave the project of finding a cure for migraine to the unfettered enterprise of all these separate individual inclinations to keep trying – joined, of course, by all those medical entrepreneurs who will service the inclination – there is at least a logical possibility we may finally stumble on something that is safe and effective. Our *practical* chances of success are, however, enormously improved if we *organize* our effort to find a migraine cure around the established system of experimentation that is used by medical science. Bringing effective social organization to such a scientific effort means, however, that the ordinary freedom of persons to keep trying therapies will be limited. Getting organized translates into getting governed.

Rational migraine sufferers have to weigh the relative attractiveness of two scenarios: one in which they have a completely privatized and unfettered right to scour the earth for novel therapies for their affliction, and in which they have virtually no practical chance of success; and another in which they must relinquish a measure of their therapeutic autonomy to a social and scientific authority that will organize the search for a cure according to the scientific method. The latter, scientific scenario is the easy winner in this contest. Of course, it suffers from the fault of being a choice that entails a measure of paternalism. But we have, in this connection as in the instance of general consumer interests, historically accepted a very limited paternalism because of the substantial benefits gained through its narrow operation. A nation without migraine is a better nation, and it is especially a better nation for migraine sufferers – which is one good reason, among several others, that we don't hear cries of 'human guinea pigs!' in protest at controlled investigation of experimental headache cures.

The point to be taken from all this is that the regulation of drugs isn't just an authoritative whim or bad habit of government. It is grounded in, and legitimized by, the effort to protect public health. In the case of the Canadian regulatory authority – the federal Health Protection Branch – there is an additional historical backdrop to its austere scientific conservatism. In the early 1960s, it approved the notorious morning-sickness drug Thalidomide. Payment of damages to the victims of that drug's toxic effects on embryos was recently offered by the federal government, but the aftershocks of the Thalidomide disaster have been institutionalized in the stubborn resistance, on the part of the officials of the HPB, to liberalization of the regulatory process. If federal bureaucracies are ever issued with heraldic coats of arms, the Branch's will certainly bear the emblem '*Once Burned* . . . '. Ironically, the American counterpart of the HPB, the Federal Drug Agency, has drawn the same conservative lesson from the Thalidomide episode, even though it covered itself in glory by blocking the sale of the drug. For the FDA, the motto – pressed into service as the unanswerable justification for every instance of regulatory strictness – would be: '*We Saved You From Thalidomide*'.

ANOTHER KINGDOM

The clear statement of a public interest is usually sufficient to set aside the interested claims of individuals; but to think it must *always* be so is an error grounded in the confusion of interests with rights. In our moral and legal tradition, some individual interests are given a special status as *rights* that *may* act as political 'trumps' over ordinarily dominant public interests – to use the felicitous expression introduced by Ronald Dworkin.[6]

For example, it is rumoured that a certain Third World Communist country tests experimental vaccines for catastrophic illnesses on those of its prison population convicted of political offences. Efficacy tests of vaccines are notoriously difficult when investigators are limited to the statistical study of voluntary subjects over a period of time long enough to yield significant results. The scientific virtues of simply injecting live pathogens into vaccinated subjects and observing the outcome are obvious, as are the public interests served by doing effective science quickly rather than slowly. But Canadians are appalled by any such policy, discovering in its simplistic weighing of public against individual interests a tyrannical disregard for the *rights* of the coerced experimental subjects. I offer this example not as a pretended analogy to the issue before us, but rather to engage, with an extreme case, our relevant moral intuitions about the special significance of individual rights.

What rights claims can PLWAs fairly make? First of all, that the catastrophically ill are set apart from the general patient population by the fact that they face, in addition to the suffering ordinarily associated with illness, the ultimate human disaster of death. *No human crisis more powerfully concentrates a claim to self-determination in the hands of individuals than does their impending death.* Second, they can claim that competence is a necessary condition for the justification of any paternalistic system. After all, it is because 'Father knows best' that he has both the right and the duty to limit the freedom of his children 'for their own sake'; and it is because established medicine knows best how to treat sickness that it has an authoritative role to play in governing therapy. But, by the same token and logic, where the therapeutic system must admit a lack of competence, it should also admit that its ordinary authority is compromised or weakened. The catastrophically ill are, as it were, perched on a crumbling ledge over a chasm. No establishment-certified ropes can reach them, so the therapeutic authorities have less justification for limiting the freedom of such patients to try to save themselves with their own choice of unapproved rope.

Indeed, the loneliness of the catastrophically ill, relegated to Another Kingdom by our powerlessness to reach out to them with curative hope, calls to mind the situation of that other medical loner, the patient who refuses treatment. The right to refuse even established therapy is perhaps the most settled feature of patients' rights in the democracies. It is clearly rooted in the importance of individual integrity in our scheme of things, and the correlative right guaranteed to an individual adult to 'secure his person' by his or her own lights and in his or her own way. Indeed, we have almost a horror of the imposition of medical treatment, however well-intentioned, as a palpable invasion of personal integrity. It offends our basic intuitions concerning both the foundations and the objects of democratic life.

There is a significant symmetry between the well-established right of the 'refusing' patient and the novel claim for catastrophic rights. It rests in the conflict, in both instances, between an individual patient's vision of what is best for himself or herself – rooted in a personal conception of what is requisite to the maintenance of his or her life, or a religious conviction, or even a determination to die – and society's vision of what is generally best for everyone. And in both cases, the patient appeals to the special importance we attach to, and the special rights we provide for, the self-determination of individuals in that which affects them most personally and profoundly.

There are, of course, asymmetries between these two rights, most significantly that the refusing patient demands nothing, while the catastrophic patient demands something that is in the gift of others. The difference and gap are, however, significantly narrowed when we recognize that what each patient confronts is the same social and political entity – the therapeutic authorities – to which society has granted practically absolute powers over the development of medicines and the treatment of disease. The decision to honour the refusal of treatment, or permit treatment with one drug but not with another, or to forbid treatment with the patient's choice of therapy, has, by becoming a social prerogative, become a social responsibility. In our system, such social authority may be curbed or limited by the legitimate claim of an individual right, and it is from this perspective that catastrophic-rights claims are made.

To the extent to which there is symmetry between the circumstances of the refusing and the catastrophic patient, there ought also to be symmetry between the individual rights accorded them as against *ordinarily* overriding public interests. These rights should be, at a conservative minimum, as broad as possible to reflect our respect for self-determination in that which affects an individual most personally and profoundly, and as narrow as is necessary to leave materially undisturbed the *vital* public health interests sought through the social control of therapies. In this spirit, I turn now to a consideration of the application of such rights to the special case for governmental regulation of *catastrophic* drugs.

Paternalism revisited. While the paternalistic governance of therapies may well make moral and legal sense in the case of ordinary illnesses, thwarting the deliberate therapeutic choices of the catastrophically ill flies in the face of the universal moral intuition that dying people ought to have more than an ordinary say in how they play their (last) cards. If we recognize a catastrophic right of *symmetrical* force and limits with the right to refuse treatment – that is, with the same narrow range of possible consequences for persons other than the patient – then whatever justification we may have for limiting the therapeutic autonomy of the catastrophically ill, it cannot be that we thwart them 'for their own good'. Whatever their claim to be the best judges of their own interests, there can be no question that their extreme personal danger enhances their *right* to assess and take their own therapeutic risks.

This raises a troubling set of considerations for physicians. Physicians have a professional obligation to avoid causing harm to their patients. How can they discharge this obligation when they are asked to co-operate in the acquisition and administration of unapproved drugs, the safety and efficacy of which are scientific question marks? My view of this is that the professional responsibility to avoid harm must be assessed within a broad – as opposed to a narrow – conception of the patient's welfare. For instance, and just to make the principle clear with a limiting case, many of us would deny, as a categorical limitation governing the provision of medical care, the rule that a physician cannot be involved in active euthanasia. Given a range of procedural protections, which I need not detail here, many of us would regard a physician as professionally correct in acceding to the clear request of an adult, competent, terminal patient for help in ending his or her life with dignity. Now, the causing of death is ordinarily thought of as a very great – if not the greatest – harm that can be done to a human being. But in the case of euthanasia, we recognize that the refusal of a physician to take into consideration the deliberate and clearly stated desire of a patient is to refuse to accept, as a highly relevant factor in determining the patient's welfare, the patient's own personal assessment of how he or she wishes to spend his life; and to do so is to visit a real harm upon the patient.

The general point I want to make here is that the deliberate therapeutic choices of patients must be carefully figured into any professional assessment of what is in their welfare. Human beings have bodies – but to insist that persons are *only* flesh and blood would make even their clear *refusal* of treatment an irrelevant consideration.

So when we consider the ethical concerns of medical professionals in connection with their co-operation in the provision of catastrophic therapies, our attention should centre on the intentionality of their patients' therapeutic choices. Are the patients reasonably well-informed? Do they understand the full range of possible consequences of the choice of an inadequately tested therapy? Have they been given a clear, complete, and objective account of their prognosis – with all of the uncertain positive as well as negative possibilities? If these matters have been professionally attended to, and the patients clearly and unequivocally elect to try a catastrophic therapy, they are giving a very clear indication of how they choose to spend their life. To thwart them may, possibly, buy them extra time; but, by definition, it is most improbable that it can save them from their catastrophic prognosis. The refusal to recognize such patients' catastrophic right to try an untested therapy is based upon a narrow, and hence incorrect, assessment of the patients' welfare.

It is here that the distinction between the non-catastrophic versus catastrophic situation comes into sharp focus. For if the illness under consideration were migraine rather than AIDS, I would remain convinced of the merits of the case made out earlier for the social control of therapy. But a catastrophic situation undercuts the general case for medical paternalism, because established medicine is simply without the means to guarantee that if it thwarts catastrophic patients' therapeutic wishes, its doing so will result in 'their own good'. A catastrophic illness has a levelling influence on the relative claims to therapeutic competence of the physician and patient, and this justifies such patients' claim to a greater measure of self-determination in their treatment.

This does *not* mean that physicians are always wrong to refuse to participate in the administration of an unapproved treatment. Physicians are the professional allies of their patients, not their creatures; respect for the catastrophic rights of patients doesn't translate into abandoning them to 'pick their own poison'. My point is, rather, that in arriving at their professional judgements, physicians should give respectful consideration to the informed, deliberate, and clearly stated therapeutic choices of their patients. These choices should be attended to not as something *extrinsic* to the professional medical task, but rather as an *intrinsic* element of any adequate assessment of the patient's welfare, as this serves the correlative goal of avoiding harm.

Conservation of limited health-care resources revisited. As in the case of the ordinary arguments in support of medical paternalism, catastrophic illness presents us with exceptional circumstances when we turn to the issue of cost-effectiveness. It is clear that governing the administration of therapies – 'You may take this medicine; you may not take that' – is *positively* related to the conservation of health-care resources in the case of the *non*-catastrophically ill. The sooner we make this class of patients well, the sooner they will no longer be drawing on our resources. But the catastrophically ill are dying, and dying because medical science is powerless to save them. As the warning posters in the bars of Bangkok starkly state: 'AIDS YOU DIE. NO CURE.' In the face of this, the only reasonable near-term claim that can be made, in 1990, for limiting the therapeutic freedom of the catastrophically ill is that such a restriction *may* prevent them from dying sooner as the consequence of an unsuccessful gamble on an unproven treatment. But whatever the positive *protective* consequences of such medical paternalism, it has negative *economic* consequences. This is because of a grim axiom of medical economics: next to a patient who is very quickly cured, the cheapest patient to treat is one who is very quickly dead.

But what about the long term? We have noted that one of the arguments for sacrificing individual autonomy to those public interests connected with the claims of science focuses on the consideration that if we do so we will be able to offer safer, more effective, and hence more *economical* treatments to future patients. But just as this is probably a good bet, it is an even better bet that those 'better' treatments will not be, in the case of AIDS, *cheaper*, or treatments that husband our limited health-care resources. They will be the most expensive treatments imaginable in the case of a catastrophic illness, the kind that buy time and comfort without curing. When the going gets tough for medical science – which is, by definition, the general case with the catastrophic illnesses – even 'dramatic' progress is measured incrementally. Thus one of the comments that can be made with confidence about the strengths and weaknesses of modern medical science is that, with but few extraordinary exceptions, they are perfectly balanced to generate remarkably expensive standards of treatment for serious illnesses in general, and catastrophic illnesses in particular. Doubts on this head can be resolved by considering the health-care costs associated with the present regimen of treatments for the cancers.

The protection of science revisited. Even though society doesn't have a good public-interest argument to justify limiting catastrophic rights for paternalistic or economic reasons, it still has a case for doing so, in the case of AIDS at least, that is rooted in the most fundamental of public health concerns – the control of *infectious* deadly disease. More than anything else, it is the infectious character of AIDS that makes scientific progress everybody's business. A fair statement of society's case for exercising a therapeutic authority that limits the catastrophic rights of PLWAs would then, at this point in our discussion, go something like this: 'Let's say that we give you the ground we previously claimed for paternalistic or economic reasons. That gives a certain force and range to your idea of catastrophic rights, but still leaves us occupying some territory that we cannot responsibly surrender to you. We cannot abandon our efforts to make scientific headway against your disease, because we have an obligation to protect the health of all of society from infection with it, and we have a related obligation to make such progress for the sake of those who may not have your disease now, but who will certainly get it and suffer your fate if we cannot discover a cure or more effective treatments. We have, in a manner of speaking, a "practice" that extends beyond you to those who are at risk now, and those who *will* fall ill in the future. Thus your voluntary participation (which is also your vote of confidence in medical science) in our controlled trials of therapies for your illness must continue to be governed by us. Only in that way can we protect our ability to do science, and thus provide for a range of health interests that extends beyond yours. These public health interests are vital, and must be pursued no matter what the costs, either to individuals whose freedom is thereby restricted, or to society, whose treasure is expended.'

SCIENCE AND RIGHTS

This brings us to the heart of the public-interest argument for limiting the therapeutic autonomy of the catastrophically ill; and it is a strong argument. This is not, however, a case of the civil-rights cow that gives a full pail of milk, only to kick it over when frightened by a public interest. Strong does not mean absolute. It means, rather, that while there is a *vital* public-interest case for limiting catastrophic rights, it can justify only limitations of such rights as will materially advance the achievement of the *specific and vital* public health goal of protecting the ability of medical science to find an effective cure or treatment for AIDS. Only that public purpose is sufficiently compelling and, presumably, attainable – at least in the eyes of everyone affected – to prevail against the claim of an individual catastrophic right.

In this connection it is important to remember that although individual interests must ordinarily give way to public interests, individual rights ordinarily should not. One properly speaks of individual *interests* being balanced against competing public interests: but individual *rights* are not balanced against ordinary public interests – they override them. This refers to the 'trumping' character of rights, which was mentioned earlier. However, when we identify an extraordinary public interest – one that is vital and compelling – the trumping force of competing individual rights is lessened, though the situation is then not as simple as one of public interest holding sway over private interest.

An example may help. The Second Section of the Canadian Charter of Rights and Freedoms and the First Amendment of the US Constitution identify the intellectual freedoms of thought and expression as the bedrock individual rights of democracy. We will insist upon these rights even when their exercise directly conflicts with an important public interest such as the maintenance of loyal respect for our form of government. The lesson of the McCarthy era in the US – or what the American journalist I.F. Stone called the 'haunted Fifties' – was that even Marxist calls for our governments to be smashed, and their officials liquidated, must not be prohibited or limited by law. Imagine, however, a Marxist pamphlet containing plans that would make it possible for anyone with fifty dollars and a few simple tools to make a crude atomic bomb. We would certainly, and correctly, prohibit the publication of such a pamphlet as representing an extraordinary threat to a set of public interests properly described as 'vital'. We can argue with the Marxists about how we should, or should not, organize our political lives; but argument cannot save us from wholesale slaughter if the power to destroy entire cities is brought within the independent means of anybody and everybody. The logic of the situation is then, in a manner of speaking, that society itself faces a catastrophic situation, and its corporate catastrophic right to protect the conditions for its survival override the ordinarily trumping force of rights. Even such a vital public interest would not legitimize, however, the prohibition of *all* Marxist pamphlets; it could only justify the censorship of pamphlets that contained the cheap bomb plans.

My point here is that an individual right continues to have significance even when its trumping force is overridden by a public interest that is vital and compelling. A right overridden does not shrink into a mere interest; it continues to exert a shaping, cautionary pressure on policy. Our moral and legal culture has developed several general ruling considerations that apply in such circumstances.

First, the right should be overridden only so far as is necessary in order to address the *vital and compelling* character of the competing public interest. Ordinary public interests do not avail against the expression of a genuine right. Thus if a *proportional*, or partial, approach for the protection of the vital public interest is possible, it should be vigorously explored. In practical terms, this simply means that the state should always try to preserve a right intact; and where it can't, it should cut into the right only so far as is absolutely necessary.

Second, since the right is being overridden in order to provide for a specific vital public interest, the limitations imposed must be *specific* rather than general. A case for the limitation of catastrophic rights that rests upon the vital public interest in finding a cure for AIDS cannot serve as an umbrella under which the therapeutic authorities can limit catastrophic rights for (plausible) other reasons – usually paternalistic or economic ones.

Finally, the claim of the existence of a public interest that is so vital and compelling as to legitimize the setting aside of an individual right places an obligation upon the state with respect to *performance*. A public interest retains its status as vital or compelling – and hence legitimately continues to out-weigh individual rights claims – just in case government's regard for it as such is validated by the efforts actually made to attain it. There is, of course, no cut and dried way of determining whether government is exerting itself in such a way as sustains the claim that it is seriously and responsibly pursuing an interest it regards as vital. Nonetheless, we should accept the principle that just as there is a difference between interests that are vital and those that are merely 'nice to have', there is also a discernible difference in the behaviour of individuals and governments as they seek to provide for one or the other.

DOING THE RIGHT THING

In the final analysis, choosing to submit to randomization in a classically controlled experiment involves a limited personal sacrifice of autonomy. The scope of such sacrifice can, however, be significantly reduced by the specific care that is brought to the design of the experiment. Within the 'envelope' of scientifically sound investigation, everyone recognizes that experimental design can be wasteful of time, material, professional talent, or even human lives. *It can also be wasteful of the therapeutic autonomy of its subjects.* Recognition of this fact, conjoined with respect for catastrophic rights, should motivate an effort to trim away both the material and the conceptual fat from formal trials of catastrophic therapies.

Like economies, experimental designs can be expected to respond more speedily and flexibly to ideals that are joined to a range of tolerable pressures than to ideals alone. As long as catastrophic subjects can be recruited on a 'take it or leave it' basis (where 'take it' entails submitting to randomization and surrendering a significant measure of therapeutic autonomy, and 'leave it' means no chance of getting the possibly effective experimental drug), there is little difficulty in finding subjects. Such trials have been – at least with respect to their wastefulness of patient autonomy – sloppily designed and run because, to put it baldly, they didn't have to be sold to a set of medically sophisticated prospective subjects as a rational personal option. But if patients can choose between simply obtaining a new drug in an unblinded clinical setting (an *open arm*) or becoming a subject in a formal 'gold standard' investigation of its effectiveness and safety, those who choose the trial option will be genuine volunteers, and much less likely to join the 'cheaters and rebels' who break with subject discipline. Such an arrangement would create a positive incentive to design lean, smart experiments that serve both of our relevant masters – justice for individuals, and medical progress for society. Such experiments are possible.

That possibility has been taken most seriously in Canada by Dr Martin Schechter, head of AIDS research at the University of British Columbia. Schechter has explored a range of innovative adjustments to traditional scientific practice that are responsive to catastrophic rights. For instance, on the question of error levels in determining the safety and efficacy of experimental drugs, he has said:

> These levels ought to be set based on the 'societal' costs of making false positive and false negative errors and not simply by convention. It seems ludicrous to maintain the same levels for HIV therapy trials that one would use for a trial of a lotion for mild acne. . . . We recognize a price will have to be paid in the form of increased false positive results but we believe this preferable to a state of therapeutic anarchy.[7]

In assessing the medical and public-health benefits this way, Schechter is pointing out that the smart way to approach medically sophisticated and politically determined patients is with experimental options that are sensitive to the personal realities of the catastrophically ill. Those are the only options that will be voluntarily elected, and hence the only basis for a stable program of experimentation with this subject group.

The argument against the open-arm option centres on the possibility – certainty, on some accounts – that making trials genuinely voluntary would doom controlled experimentation. The rush to the set of parallel tracks (a form of open arm) connected to the recent formal trials of the drug DDI in the US is often cited in support of this thesis, but that outcome should not be seen as a fair test of voluntarism. The inclusion criteria of the DDI trials were hopelessly restrictive to start with, and in some instances subjects would have had to have been the victims of systematic malpractice to qualify. 'For example, one of the formal studies is designed to determine whether individuals who develop anaemia taking AZT do better with DDI. To be eligible for the formal study, an individual must demonstrate that AZT has reduced the oxygen-carrying capacity of his blood by more than 40 per cent, as measured through his level of hemoglobin.'[8] American DDI researchers pointed out that most physicians would have begun blood transfusions, or stopped AZT, before such serious anaemia developed.[9]

In a sense, the anti-reform theorists admit that being a human subject in the trial of a catastrophic drug has, historically at least, been such a bad deal that nobody would consent to it if there wasn't a measure of coercion involved. In fact, when asked if they would join the trials that they are personally running, most medical professionals just say 'no'. Regulatory conservatives themselves point out, in this connection, that it is altogether natural to want to take complete control of what you are doing when faced with the danger of a catastrophic illness. The conclusion that they draw from these admissions is that we must unflinchingly, if regretfully, continue to sacrifice patient autonomy to the over-arching demands of medical progress.

Responding to the same admissions, I heartily agree with the point about catastrophic patients' wanting to take control of their own therapeutic destinies; I then insist that the therapeutic authorities get scientific about determining what can be done. There is, finally, only one way to determine if controlled experimentation on catastrophic drugs can succeed under conditions of genuine voluntarism, and that is to give it an earnest try. Whether it can work is an empirical question, and such questions ought not be prejudged when important rights issues hinge upon their answer. If our best efforts fail, it may be necessary to revisit some form of the coercive devils that we know – adjusting the voluntarist pressures on the trial system downward only as far as is demonstrably necessary in order to preserve our vital public interest in medical progress. For now, however, the therapeutic authorities should mount, as their first order of business, a vigorous, organized effort to co-ordinate our scientific agenda with the legitimate demands placed upon it by the rights of the catastrophically ill. As Schechter and others have pointed out, medical science has a lot of running room available in which to provide a far greater measure of therapeutic autonomy to its experimental subjects. It is high time that it started to use it.

Government doesn't need to apologize for governing when it is confronted with a deadly, infectious, and incurable disease. The issue is not *whether* to govern catastrophic drugs, but *how*. A doctrine of catastrophic rights is not intended, in this environment, to be a fresh thorn in the side of North American regulatory authorities. To be sure, and especially to the extent that they embody justice considerations, these rights are *for* persons living with AIDS; but they are also *for* society and its therapeutic authorities, in that they afford the possibility of replacing the endless varieties of pressure politics (which are presently threatening to cripple AIDS research) with a means of adjudicating the intensifying conflict between individual desires and public duties. When seen in this light, the recognition of these patients' rights will not disarm society's therapeutic authorities. Rather, it will provide them with a timely and legitimizing reinforcement of their traditional resources.

NOTES

[1]"Early AZT Treatment Prolongs Life', *DIMENSIONS* (7 June 1989): 3.

[2]"Conventional Use of Investigational Drugs Jeopardizing Controlled Studies', *DIMENSIONS*: 1-2.

[3]Ibid.: 1.

[4]Robert J. Levine, 'Ethicist's Role', in the 'Research for Treatments and Vaccines', colloquium of the 5th International Conference on AIDS, 7 June 1989.

[5]See, for instance, my own comments as reported in a story by Michelle Lalonde, 'People With Disease Call Use of Placebos in Drug Trials Unfair', *Globe and Mail* (8 June 1989): A12.

[6]Ronald Dworkin, *Taking Rights Seriously* (Cambridge, MA: Harvard University Press, 1977).

[7]David A. Salisbury and Martin T. Schechter, 'Aids Trials, Civil Liberties, and the Social Control of Therapy: Should We Embrace New Drugs with Open Arms?', *Canadian Medical Association Journal* 142, 2 (1990): 1057-62.

[8]As reported by Marlene Cimons in the *Los Angeles Times* (9 Nov. 1989).

[9]Ibid.

WARNING: AIDS HEALTH PROMOTION PROGRAMS MAY BE HAZARDOUS TO YOUR AUTONOMY

PATRICIA ILLINGWORTH

As of January 1990, 3,373 persons (mostly gay men and intravenous drug users) have contracted or died from AIDS in Canada.[1] HIV/AIDS challenges individuals, society, the medical sciences, and those involved in developing AIDS social policy. Applied ethicists, social-policy makers, lawyers, civil-liberties groups, and AIDS activists have struggled with the question of what measures to adopt to cope with the spread of HIV/AIDS.[2] Among the more intrusive options that have been considered (and usually rejected) are isolation, mandatory testing, and contact tracing. But if there has been widespread disagreement about the appropriateness of these measures from moral, legal, and policy perspectives, there has been consensus that education is an appropriate response to the spread of HIV/AIDS. Of the panoply of policy measures that have been considered for adoption, education programs appear to be the least intrusive; they are seen as both effective and morally praiseworthy.

The important question of whether or not the state has any business promoting some life-styles (healthy ones) over other life-styles (unhealthy ones) has been addressed elsewhere.[3] I am willing to grant, for the purposes of this paper, that the state has a legitimate role to play in the area of health education. Here my concern is not with the legitimacy of this role, but with a specific kind of health education, namely, 'health promotion', and with respect to a specific disease. In what follows I will challenge the assumption that AIDS education is morally unproblematic by considering it in the light of individual autonomy.

The crux of the problem is that some AIDS prevention programs do not, as Leroy Walters has put it, simply 'appeal to the rational capacities of the hearer'.[4] That is, they do not solely convey information on the basis of which individuals can make informed decisions about behaviour that is high-risk for HIV. These programs, which I shall refer to as 'health promotion' programs,[5] rely on manipulative techniques in order to induce people to (1) come to hold certain beliefs and, as a result, to (2) change their unhealthy behaviour. From the point of view of respect for autonomy, programs that employ manipulative techniques, even in the service of a good end – such as a long and healthy life – are problematic.

This paper is divided into three parts. In Part 1, I discuss the concepts of 'autonomy' and 'manipulation' and argue that manipulation compromises autonomy. Then, in Part 2, I show how the Canadian Public Health Association's brochure 'The New Facts of Life' is informed by manipulative techniques that violate autonomy. In Part 3, I consider whether health promotion programs that make use of manipulative techniques can be justified despite these autonomy-based objections to them. I conclude that given well-founded scepticism about their long-term effectiveness, they cannot be justified on the basis of considerations of long-term autonomy or the general welfare. Although it would be a mistake to assume that respect for individual autonomy 'trumps' all other values and in all cases, it is fair to say that the violation of individual autonomy counts as a serious shortcoming in a policy. Whether it is the decisive value in any particular case depends upon what other values are at issue and the importance ascribed to them. In this particular case, I argue that benefit to the general welfare, a potentially competing value, is not well served by AIDS health promotion programs.

PART 1

Autonomy Compromised

Before turning to an evaluation of AIDS prevention and health promotion programs, something needs to be said about respect for individual autonomy, the criterion on which this analysis is based.[6] Philosophers as diverse as Kant and Mill in the past and contemporary thinkers such as Rawls, Dworkin, and Raz have viewed autonomy as central to the moral sphere. Yet despite the importance that this concept has come to have in different moral systems, and more recently in the field of biomedical ethics, there continues to be controversy about what 'autonomy' is. This controversy cannot be settled here. What I can do, however, is to say enough about the concept for it to serve as a useful mechanism in analysing health promotion programs.

In *On Liberty*, John Stuart Mill articulated an important principle to distinguish cases of justified interference with individual freedom from cases of unjustified interference:

> As soon as any part of a person's conduct affects prejudicially the interests of others, society has jurisdiction over it, and the question whether the general welfare will or will not be promoted by interfering with it, becomes open to discussion. But there is no room for entertaining any such question when a person's conduct affects the interests of no persons besides himself, or needs not affect them unless they like. . . . In all such cases there should be perfect freedom, legal and social, to do the action and stand the consequences.[7]

According to Mill's harm principle, interference in a person's freedom of action is justified when the action to be interfered with harms other people and the interference promotes the general welfare. Actions that harm only the person who performs them cannot be interfered with solely on the grounds that such interference is in the best interest of the agent. This principle is grounded on the importance assigned to preserving a sphere of freedom in which people can conduct their lives as they see fit. What speaks for preserving such a sphere is that people, unlike most other animals, have a capacity to reflect, to make choices, and to act on their choices. Mill also believed that individuals are themselves in the best position to determine their best interest.[8]

In the above passage, Mill stresses the importance of being free to act as one wishes in the case of one's self-regarding actions. But the domain of human actions, understood mainly as bodily movements, is not the only domain in which people need freedom. For Mill, people's desires and impulses should also be their own: 'A person whose desires and impulses are his own – are the expression of his own nature, as it has been developed and modified by his own culture – is said to have character. One whose desires and impulses are not his own, has no character, no more than a steam engine has character.'[9] Motives, desires, wants, wishes, and impulses constitute another domain in which freedom is important. Without freedom in this domain, freedom of action would amount to very little.

Gerald Dworkin, in his most recent book, *The Theory and Practice of Autonomy*, writes that the 'idea of autonomy . . . includes . . . some ability both to alter one's actions and, indeed, to make them effective because one has reflected upon them and adopted them as one's own'.[10] Both Mill and Dworkin take the notion of 'one's own' to be central to autonomy. According to Mill it is people's desires that must be their own; according to Dworkin, their actions. Although it is not entirely clear how something comes to qualify as being 'one's own', it has something to do with an agent's reflecting on the action or desire and, in this way, coming to identify with it.[11]

Underlying Dworkin's account is the idea that in order to be autonomous, one must be able to modify one's behaviour as a result of having reflected upon it and having found that the modified behaviour is in concert with one's self. Thus autonomy also involves a capacity to reflect on one's desires and actions. Following the spirit of Dworkin's work on this topic, I shall refer to the process of reflection, and the identification with an action or desire that comes with it, as 'authenticity'. Whether an action will be 'one's own' also depends, in part, on one's projects, values, life plans, and conception of 'self'. Because actions are intimately connected with desires and beliefs, autonomy also requires that one's desires and beliefs be one's own. Thus autonomous action involves (1) acting in ways that are authentic to one's self and (2) acting in these ways because one has reflected on them and found them to be authentic or has succeeded in making them 'one's own' through reflection.

Although this account of 'autonomy' is admittedly murky, different moral virtues, such as empathy and what Bernard Williams has called the 'human point of view', bear witness to the importance we attribute to an agent's own perspective on his or her life and actions and to others' taking that perspective into consideration.[12] If people did not have a capacity to reflect on their actions and to make them their own, these virtues would be meaningless, as would the idea that we owe persons respect. But, far from being meaningless, they are at the heart of our understanding of how we ought to treat people. To fail to take into account an agent's perspective is to treat that individual as less than a person; it is to ignore the fact that his or her actions come about as a result of reflection and consideration.

In this paper our concern is with the change from unhealthy behaviour to healthy behaviour. This change can be either autonomous or non-autonomous. In order to adopt a healthy behaviour autonomously, one must adopt it only after reflecting upon it and finding it in harmony with one's self. To the extent that one's capacity to reflect on the new behaviour is undermined, so is one's autonomy. The desires that are instrumental in effecting the behaviour change should be ones with which the agent identifies.

Manipulation

There are a number of ways in which individual autonomy can be impeded. But the primary mechanism through which health promotion programs can compromise autonomy is manipulation. Joel Feinberg, in an article entitled 'Freedom and Behavior Control', gives the following account of 'manipulation':

> Manipulation of another person characteristically works directly upon his beliefs, motives, and psychological capacities and effects change neither by means of rational persuasion nor by means of external hindrances, prods and deprivations. Some forms of manipulation, for example, extortion and aversion therapy, employ threats or something very like threats and are thus properly located near the vague boundary between coercion and manipulation.[13]

When behaviour change is achieved by modifying desires, beliefs, and motives in a way that sidesteps the capacity to reflect, yet does not at the same time make use of coercive mechanisms, then the resulting behaviour is the product of manipulation. Consider an example. If people purchase a product only because barely detectable images that conjure up associations of pleasure have been placed on it as a marketing device, then their behaviour has been manipulated and their autonomy compromised. They act not as a result of their rational capacities, one of which is the capacity to reflect, but rather because their desires have been targeted by an external source. Whether by drugs, provocative images projected onto products, or strategically placed information, manipulation impedes free and unfettered decision-making. By targeting beliefs, motives, and desires, while sidestepping the capacity to reflect, manipulative techniques can modify behaviour without regard for whether the desires, impulses, and behaviour are the person's own. Behaviour that is a product of manipulation comes about despite, not because of, the person. Thus it violates autonomy.

But manipulation is not always incompatible with autonomy. When people *choose* to change their behaviour through manipulative techniques there are fewer problems for autonomy than when they are manipulated without their consent. People who, for example, choose aversion therapy in order to quit smoking subject themselves to manipulation. Here manipulation may not raise autonomy-based objections because there has been consent to the particular mechanism being used and to the goal for which it is being used.[14]

Joel Feinberg has suggested that when people freely consent to manipulation and the manipulation opens their options, autonomy-based objections to it disappear.[15] There is something to this point, but it is important to see what. Freely determined consent is important in these cases because it signals a likelihood that people *want* to change their behaviour. When we want to be manipulated into changing our behaviour, autonomy-based objections to manipulation do indeed diminish, but not because options have been increased. In this instance, manipulation facilitates realization of individuals' desires, and consent suggests that they have reflected on the desirability of the new behaviour. That is, consent functions as good grounds for believing that someone has reflected on a new behaviour.

Whether or not manipulation will enhance people's autonomy depends to some extent on whether they view the behaviour that the manipulation replaces as an impediment to their autonomy. It is worth noting here that destructive behaviour does not always qualify as an impediment to autonomy. For example, a person may see her insatiable desires as intimately connected with her conception of 'self'; she may be a Madame Bovary type, who identifies with the romanticism of all-consuming desire. Hence it is a mistake to assume that certain behaviours are in all cases impediments to autonomy. Drug addiction, alcoholism, cigarette-smoking, and behaviour that is high-risk for HIV/AIDS can be autonomous when people have reflected on these behaviours and adopted them as their own. It is therefore not safe to assume that so called 'undesirable behaviour' is always non-autonomous.

With respect to programs that manipulate individuals without their consent, individual autonomy is threatened in two distinct ways. First, these programs can saddle people with behaviour that is alien to them. Second, even when people regard the new healthy behaviour as desirable, manipulation without consent denies them an opportunity to make the new behaviour their own through reflection. That is, it denies them an important opportunity to participate wholeheartedly in their own behaviour change.

PART 2

In this section I will analyse a specific case of manipulation in a health promotion program aimed at reducing behaviour that is high-risk for HIV. This will be done in two stages. In the first, I will introduce a model of behaviour change that is widely used in health promotion. In the second, I will show how this model is put to use in AIDS prevention and health promotion with an analysis of a Canada-based AIDS brochure.

The Health Belief Model

For public health the task has been to find a mechanism that is effective in motivating people to avoid unhealthy behaviour and adopt healthy behaviour. The health-belief model (HBM) is a partial solution to this public-health goal. This model was originally developed in the 1950s by social psychologists working in the US Public Health Service in order to explain the failure of people to undertake disease-prevention measures. Since then it has been used widely as a framework for explaining and predicting people's response to health and medical care recommendations as well as for effecting behaviour change. Vaccination for influenza, screening for Tay Sachs disease, and anti-smoking programs are only a few of the health problems to have been addressed by the HBM.[16] According to this model, people are more likely to change their behaviour if they believe that (1) they are particularly vulnerable to a disease that will have (2) severe and harmful consequences for them, (in the remainder of this paper I shall refer to these as, respectively, the 'Me Belief' and the 'Die Belief'); and if they also believe that (3) a particular health action will be efficacious and (4) will not carry with it higher costs than the benefits it promises.[17] Bearing in mind Feinberg's account of manipulation, use of the HBM in health promotion qualifies as manipulative because it targets beliefs in order to change them, without appealing to a person's cognitive faculties.

One of the main inducements used by the HBM to bring people to the 'Me Belief' and the 'Die Belief' is fear. Indeed, the 'fear' strategy is so firmly entrenched in health promotion that guidelines have been developed for its effective use. The authors of one article, for example, recommend beginning with the fear-evoking message and ensuring that while the amount of fear created is great enough to ensure awareness of the potential for harm, it is not so great as to lead to denial. They also caution that the fear level should be such that it can be managed by the adoption of the healthy behaviour.[18]

The problem with such techniques is that, in attempting to manipulate people, they may threaten autonomy. When people act because they have been intimidated or threatened, the basis of their action is not reflection but fear. This is not to say that it is impossible for people who are afraid to reflect on their actions and, ultimately, act autonomously. (The extent to which fear undermines the capacity to act autonomously probably varies with the individual; some people, perhaps because of their developmental history, are no doubt more vulnerable to a diminishment in their autonomy than others.) It does, however, raise questions as to whether such manipulation can be justified. Before examining the grounds on which the autonomy objection might be overridden, let us examine one prominent Canadian AIDS prevention program in which fear-inducing strategies play a central role.

Some Examples

The AIDS Committee of Toronto has published and is involved in publishing a number of AIDS brochures that target diverse groups, including gay men, IV drug users, prostitutes, women, and members of the Black and Asian communities. Some of the brochures contain sexually explicit language and illustrations and some do not. Many of the them are aesthetically pleasing and eye-catching. One pocket-sized brochure entitled 'Your Best Bet' provides illustrations and step-by-step instructions on how to use a condom. This brochure is purely instructive, appealing to the desire to be informed, and is free of manipulative techniques.

The Canadian AIDS Society, on the other hand, an important Ottawa-based national network of different community AIDS organizations, advocates the use of manipulative techniques echoing those of the HBM. In *Safer Sex Guidelines*, the society states that it supports the model of behaviour change that 'holds that safer sex practice is achieved and maintained when a person comes to have the following five beliefs: (1) I am personally threatened by AIDS, (2) I can prevent AIDS, (3) I can manage the necessary behavior changes, (4) I can still be sexually satisfied and (5) I have peer support for this change.'[19] As the use of the word 'threatened' in the first of these shows, the society also appears to stand behind the use of fear in health promotion programs.

The Canadian Public Health Association's AIDS Education and Awareness Program publishes a newsletter and a brochure, both of which are entitled 'The New Facts of Life'.[20] These publications can easily be identified by the fear-evoking slogan 'Join the Attack on AIDS'. Like the 'War on Drugs', the CPHA's 'Attack on AIDS' campaign uses a military metaphor that carries with it a twofold message: that there is a threatening enemy (AIDS) and that this enemy must be destroyed. That the intention is to evoke fear is confirmed in the brochure, where the slogan's appearance is followed with the statement that 'AIDS is a new and frightening disease. . . '.[21] But the expression 'Join the attack on AIDS' does more than create fear: it also suggests, though no doubt unintentionally, that persons with AIDS are themselves to be attacked. But HIV/AIDS cannot be attacked in an aerial dog-fight. Instead, this 'war' is a matter of hand-to-hand combat – in which the opponent can all too easily be transformed from the invisible virus to its visible human victims. As the 'War on Drugs' has been reduced to a war on people, so the 'Attack on AIDS' may become a campaign against people who are sick with AIDS.

The slogan 'Join the Attack on AIDS' is not the only manipulative technique used in this brochure. In the main text, consisting of questions and answers, the first question raised, 'How serious is HIV infection?' is answered with 'Very serious'.[22] Following the HBM and the guidelines on the optimal use of fear, the brochure identifies HIV as a serious harm (in this way fostering the 'Die Belief') and commences with the fear-inducing message. The next question, 'How do *you* become infected with HIV?', is answered with a list of six behaviours that can spread HIV.[23] Printed in bold type is the following:

> *Sexual Intercourse*: Any person infected with HIV can transmit the virus to another person through sexual activity where semen, vaginal fluids, or blood enter the other person's body. Vaginal intercourse and anal intercourse are the highest risk activities; oral sex may also be risky.[24]

Although it is not inaccurate to say that vaginal and anal intercourse are 'the highest risk activities', it is misleading to couple them in this way, because there is good evidence that the risk with anal intercourse is significantly higher than with vaginal intercourse. It is not difficult to explain why anal and vaginal intercourse have been treated as alike in this respect if we are mindful of the HBM. The question to which this concatenation is a response is 'How do *you* become infected?' To put vaginal intercourse in perspective would have diminished the extent to which people who have *exclusively* vaginal intercourse would believe themselves to be susceptible to HIV disease: these people (not an insignificant number) would not come to hold the 'Me Belief' and if the HBM is right, they would therefore be less likely to change their behaviour.

The next question, 'What does *not* cause infection?', and the answer to it seem to function as a way of dissipating the fear introduced earlier in the brochure. The answer begins with an encouraging statement – 'The good news is that HIV infection cannot be caught through casual everyday contact' – and continues with a list of everyday activities that are not risky for HIV. This section works with the previous one to suggest that individuals can control whether or not they come into contact with HIV. Knowing which activities transmit the disease and which do not helps to foster belief (3) of the HBM, that a particular health action will be efficacious. If HIV could be transmitted through casual contact as well as high-risk behaviour, low-risk behaviour would seem to be pointless.

Fear, however, is triggered again with the question 'Is there a treatment for HIV infection?' and the response that at present there is no cure, and that those who have HIV disease 'face a difficult life battle'.[25] The message that HIV is a serious disease about which a person should be concerned is repeated, again with a military metaphor. But this fear is ignited only to be extinguished in the next two pages of the brochure, where the question 'How can you protect yourself from infection?' is raised and answered with the following four recommendations: (1) Choose one uninfected partner for life; (2) Practise safer sex; (3) Use only latex rubber condoms; and (4) Avoid intravenous drug use.[26] These are feasible behaviour options.

Yet other options are excluded. For example, people could have been informed of the option of abstaining from sexual intercourse altogether and instead enjoying frottage and mutual masturbation. Furthermore, if people are not going to incorporate safer sex practices into their sexual repertoire, they could be discouraged from having sex in major urban centres, which have a high concentration of HIV. Lesbianism might also have been suggested as a low-risk practice. I include these options here not in order to recommend them, but only to point out that a selection has been made. Again, the HBM can be helpful by explaining the principle on which this selection is founded. Including the options I have suggested would have been counter-productive because they would strike many people as unrealizable. And if people view the behaviour changes necessary to avoid AIDS as implausible, given their other preferences, they are less likely to come to hold belief (4) – that a particular health action will not carry with it higher costs than the benefits it promises – than if they believe that the changes are feasible. Given the anxiety and fear that have been aroused by the brochure, the selection of behaviour changes that have been identified as low-risk will be seen by many people as feasible.

One explanation for the lack of more specific information might be that considerations of expense and design limited the number of questions that could be raised and answered in the brochure. It is difficult, however, to justify this explanation in view of the repetition of the uninformative slogan 'Join the attack on AIDS'. Clear and unambiguous information would seem to have been sacrificed to the goal of behaviour modification.

To entitle this brochure 'The New Facts of Life' is to present it as purely informative material that is designed to cater to the rational faculties. Yet it goes beyond the presentation of information; 'The New Facts of Life' presents the facts (and misrepresents them) in a manner designed to evoke fear and establish beliefs that, according to the HBM, will lead to the adoption of practices that are low-risk for HIV. The lavish use of military metaphor leaves little doubt that fear-evoking messages are an integral component of the brochure. The use of manipulation to establish beliefs that will foster low-risk behaviour violates individual autonomy by sidestepping people's capacity to reflect carefully and to assess their behaviour in the light of the facts.

This autonomy-based objection to 'The New Facts of Life' brochure, and others like it, might be objected to on the grounds that although manipulation occurs, there is consent to it; the argument goes as follows. In so far as its title reflects the content of a publication, people who pick up such a brochure are aware of the material contained in it; thus they consent to manipulation. Although this argument might be true in some cases, in this particular case the title 'The New Facts of Life' misleads people into believing that they are receiving purely informative material. To secure consent, this brochure would have to be identified as manipulative. For instance, it might carry a warning analogous to the one placed on cigarette packages: 'The Canadian Philosophical Association has determined that this brochure contains manipulative techniques that are hazardous to your autonomy.'[27] With such a warning, people could make informed decisions about whether they wish to subject themselves to manipulative techniques in order to modify their behaviour.

This analysis of AIDS prevention and health promotion programs in Canada is far from comprehensive; my purpose is only to establish that manipulative techniques have been employed here. To be fair to these programs, the use of manipulative techniques is by no means unique to them, nor is the example that has been discussed here the worst case of manipulation in health promotion programs. (That dubious honour may well belong to Australia's 'Grim Reaper' campaign.[28]) The organizations and government offices mentioned here offer other brochures and health-promotion programs that do not rely on manipulative techniques, and even those criticized here may be praiseworthy on grounds other than respect for autonomy – grounds that might override autonomy considerations. Some of these other considerations will now be looked at.

PART 3
Unfulfilled Promises and Unforeseen Consequences

The autonomy considerations that I have raised speak against using manipulative techniques. Yet autonomy considerations are not the only ones that are relevant to determining whether AIDS prevention and health promotion programs that make use of manipulative techniques ought to be adopted. Other criteria, such as the general welfare, should also be taken into account. Furthermore, one might argue that, from a long-term perspective, autonomy considerations speak for manipulation. According to this line of reasoning, although manipulative techniques fail to respect the autonomy of individuals at the time that manipulation takes place, by extending life they preserve autonomy over the long term. Long-term autonomy should trump short-term autonomy. For both this argument and any general-welfare-based argument to work, however, it must be the case, at the very least, that manipulative techniques are effective not only at initiating behaviour change, but also at maintaining it. Since short-term behaviour change is not enough to slow the spread of HIV, the long-term effectiveness of manipulative techniques must be addressed. Unfortunately, there is evidence to suggest that programs that make use of manipulative techniques are not particularly effective over the long term.

Healthy behaviours that carry immediate benefits for the person who practises them are self-reinforcing. For example, patient compliance with self-medication programs is high when the medication brings immediate relief from symptoms. The rewards make the healthy behaviour relatively easy to maintain.[29]

Yet this is not true for all behaviour change. Some unhealthy behaviour offers pleasure, 'stimulation and comfort' and its absence is associated with 'denial, sacrifice, withdrawal, fatigue, or some combination of these'.[30] Cigarette-smoking is a good example of an unhealthy behaviour that is pleasurable to the smoker, the cessation of which may be identified with unpleasant sensations. Furthermore, the rewards of abstaining from nicotine are remote and indirect. Behaviour change of this kind is difficult to maintain because the rewards of maintaining it are, at best, ambiguous and distant. To counteract the discouraging effects of the absence of internal rewards, health educators have created external sources of motivation and reinforcement. Among these are peer influence, tax incentives, insurance premium reductions, threat of job loss, and family and employer support.[31]

The use of external incentives is not without its own problems. To be successful at maintaining the behaviour change, the external rewards must be continuous. According to one study, 'successfully reinforced behavior becomes isolated and dependent on external reinforcement or extrinsic rewards. . . . When an individual perceives the reward as coming from sources that are distant, unconcerned, or unreliable, the behavior becomes highly contingent on the visibility and immediacy of the reward.'[32] In other words, to maintain behaviour change that has been externally motivated, the external factors that initiate it must also be maintained. In contrast, behaviour change that is founded on an individual's values is likely to be more enduring.

Before continuing, it is important to recognize that the behaviour that is high-risk for HIV/AIDS often has a significant place in the lives of those who engage in it. IV drug-use can function as a kind of solace for the poor and disinherited, and needle-sharing can serve as a bonding mechanism among members of the drug sub-culture.[33] Sexual activity, gay and straight, is a natural and important part of people's lives, and condom use is widely viewed as an impediment to pleasurable sensations. Furthermore, frequent impersonal sex, though controversially identified as high-risk, serves a variety of needs for the people who engage in it.[34]

The behaviour change that is required to lower a person's risk for HIV is not self-reinforcing. Frequent anonymous sex, sex without a condom, and the bonding connected with needle-sharing carry associations of pleasure and comfort. Abstaining from these activities will be viewed by many people as a sacrifice, the rewards of which are distant. The behaviour change that is required to slow the spread of HIV is the least susceptible to external reinforcements. Yet AIDS health promotion programs that make use of manipulative techniques rely on external reinforcements such as fear and peer pressure. Furthermore, they are likely to be viewed by many of those whom they target as remote and unconcerned, if not downright antagonistic. If this analysis is right, then programs that rely on manipulative techniques to initiate behaviour change must be continuous in order to maintain that change. In other words, long-term behaviour change requires constant exposure to manipulation. Hence it is difficult to see how manipulative techniques can promise to enhance autonomy over the long term.

Health promotion programs that attempt to diminish the spread of HIV through the use of external factors, such as manipulation, may be effective at achieving short-term behaviour change. It is not clear that they are effective at maintaining behaviour change. But if they fail over the long term, when long-term behaviour change is what is required to slow the spread of HIV, it is difficult to justify them.

In response to this, one might argue that even though health promotion programs cannot ensure long-term change, people who have been subjected to them are not any worse off than they were prior to the use of manipulative techniques. In addition to the violation to autonomy, however, there may be another harm that is not immediately obvious. Recall that the Canadian AIDS Society advocates peer support for those trying to adopt low-risk behaviour. The authors of the above study are concerned that peer support is little more than a euphemism for 'social pressure' amounting to 'nagging, harassing, badgering, or at best cajoling subjects to change their behaviour'.[35] Efforts to induce behaviour change that is not in line with a person's conception of 'self' may be not only ineffectual, but actually counter-productive. Consider the following:

> One danger of modifying behavior against the grain of the individual's own values or beliefs is that the individual left to his or her own devices will tend to rationalize why the behavior cannot be maintained and will be that much more resistant to subsequent behavioral change interventions. It produces, in short, a kind of inoculation against subsequent efforts to change the behavior by building and strengthening the individual's arguments against it.[36]

By fostering the development of arguments and defences, attempts to induce people to change their high-risk behaviour when they themselves do not wish to do so may actually diminish the likelihood that they will be able to modify their behaviour in future; their ability to adopt low-risk behaviour through more effective methods may be undermined. If this is so, then people are harmed in another way. Constant exposure to manipulation and peer pressure may stand in the way of coming to have a desire of one's own for low-risk behaviour, an authentic desire that might ultimately be more successful in ensuring long-term behaviour change. Thus AIDS prevention programs that employ manipulative techniques may undermine the very end that they seek.

If our interest is in securing autonomy over the long term, by securing a longer life span, it is not clear that the violation of short-term autonomy by manipulative techniques can be justified. Furthermore, even if we grant, as some would have it, that autonomy is not the most important value to be secured here, it is still difficult to see how we can justify violating it for what amounts to, at the best, an unclear benefit, and at the worst, a counter-productive outcome. In any case, the burden of justification falls on those who wish to violate autonomy for the sake of such uncertain goals.

Other plausible goods, such as the general welfare, that might justify the violation to autonomy inherent in manipulative programs cannot be invoked in this case, because it is not clear how these techniques can secure them. If manipulative techniques cannot slow the spread of HIV/AIDS, it is not clear that they will promote the general welfare.

It might be argued that it is not unethical to use manipulative techniques in the case of HIV/AIDS, even though they violate autonomy, because high-risk actions are not self-regarding and therefore are not protected by the harm principle. According to this reasoning, the state can invoke manipulative techniques on behalf of those who would be harmed by people who are HIV-positive. I have argued elsewhere, as have others, that the transmission of HIV falls most clearly into the harm-to-self category.[37] But it is not necessary to rehearse those arguments here in order to meet the above objection.

For Mill, interference with other people's actions, even their other-regarding actions, is not justifiable solely on the grounds that they are other-regarding. The interference must be shown to promote the general welfare. In so far as manipulative techniques are ineffective at maintaining behaviour change, they will not promote the general welfare, and therefore cannot be defended by way of the harm principle. Moreover, even if they were effective at slowing the spread of HIV/AIDS, they may entail other costs that would not promote the general welfare.

A study conducted by Robert Allard, a Montreal-based epidemiologist, showed that among the married and less-educated members of his sample there was a correlation between (1) holding the 'Me Belief' and the 'Die Belief' with respect to HIV/AIDS and (2) supporting coercive measures for persons with AIDS under epidemic conditions.[38] Thus use of the HBM in health promotion may indirectly generate support for more restrictive policies, such as quarantine.

It is also possible that the widespread fear, contempt, and hatred that have been shown towards people with HIV/AIDS can be partially explained by the campaign to establish the 'Me Belief' and the 'Die Belief' with respect to AIDS. If so, then health promotion programs may also be accountable for the lack of compassion that many persons with AIDS have faced.

This indirect consequence of the HBM must be taken into account in evaluating the consequences of the use of the HBM for the general welfare. The idea that policies and state interventions can be useful in fostering certain values is not new. In *The Gift Relationship*, Richard Titmuss defends a purely voluntary blood donor system, in part, on the grounds that it encourages, as an indirect consequence, the virtue of altruism.[39] Whether or not one agrees with the contentious assumption that the state ought to cultivate virtues in its citizens, it is important to acknowledge that the altruism for which Titmuss is arguing is a widely recognized virtue. The same cannot be said of the belief that people with AIDS ought to be quarantined – that is, incarcerated. Though many people do indeed hold such a belief, and perhaps as an indirect consequence of health promotion programs, this is by no means a widely acknowledged virtue.

Health promotion programs aimed at modifying behaviour that is high-risk for HIV/AIDS fail to respect individual autonomy. Autonomy considerations alone are not, however, enough to justify abandoning these programs. Were health promotion programs among the most effective means of initiating and maintaining behaviour change, a sacrifice to autonomy might well be warranted. Such benefit to the general welfare is an important consideration to take into account. But health promotion programs do not appear to be an especially effective mechanism through which to modify behaviour. Not only is there evidence that programs that rely on external reinforcements, such as fear and peer pressure, are not effective in maintaining behaviour change, but there is also evidence that these programs create a climate that is intolerant to persons who have HIV/AIDS.

NOTES

This article was written during a leave of absence that I had the good fortune to spend as a Senior Ethics Fellow in the Program in Psychiatry and the Law of Harvard Medical School. I wish to thank Tom Gutheil, Michael Commons, and members of the Program for providing me with important insights and a context in which to complete this work. I also wish to thank McGill University for a much needed leave of absence. An early version of this paper was presented at the 5th International Conference on AIDS. I am grateful to those who gave me comments at the conference. Many people provided me with valuable research material. Two student assistants, Harold Wilson and Nathaniel Hupert, were of help in this respect, as was Ed Jackson. I thank them. I wish also to express my gratitude to Christine Overall both for encouraging me to develop the ideas contained in this paper and for careful and thought-provoking comments about them. Many thanks go to Bill Zion as well. Finally, special appreciation should go to Harold Bursztajn, with whom I have had lengthy discussions about the ideas and arguments contained in this paper.

1 Ontario Ministry of Health, 'AIDS Statistics for Ontario and Canada' (15 Jan. 1990).

2 For a chronicle of the US debates about AIDS policy see Ronald Bayer, *Private Acts, Social Consequences: AIDS and the Politics of Public Health* (New York: The Free Press, 1989).

3 See Daniel Wickler, 'Persuasion and Coercion for Health: Ethical Issues in Government Efforts to Change Life-styles', *Milbank Memorial Fund Quarterly/Health and Society* 56, 3 (1978): 303-38. There are also interesting questions to be asked about whether the state can justifiably try to modify behaviour that is other-regarding. The important and morally relevant distinction between punishment and rehabilitation is relevant to this question.

4 Leroy Walters, 'Ethical Issues in the Prevention and Treatment of HIV Infection and AIDS', *Science* 239 (February 1988): 597-603.

5 The distinction that I draw between 'health promotion' and 'health education' is not one that appears in public health literature, where the two terms are used interchangeably.

6 For good discussions of the concept of 'autonomy' see Gerald Dworkin, *The Theory and Practice of Autonomy* (Cambridge: Cambridge University Press, 1988) and Lawrence Haworth, *Autonomy: An Essay in Philosophical Psychology and Ethics* (New Haven: Yale University Press, 1986).

7 John Stuart Mill, 'On Liberty', in *Three Essays*, introduction by Richard Wollheim (Oxford: Oxford University Press, 1975), p. 93.

8 Ibid., pp. 102-3.

9 Ibid., pp. 74-5.

10 Dworkin, p. 17.

11 For a more extensive discussion of this notion of 'autonomy' see Dworkin, pp. 3-20.

12 Bernard Williams, 'The Idea of Equality', in *Problems of the Self* (Cambridge: Cambridge University Press, 1973), pp. 230-49.

13 Joel Feinberg, 'Behavior Control: Freedom and Behavior Control', *Encyclopedia of Bioethics*, vol. 1 (New York: The Free Press, 1978), p. 97.

14 For our purposes we do not have to settle the question of whether there are autonomy-based objections to manipulation to which people consent. Certainly there are fewer autonomy-based objections to manipulation to which people consent than to manipulation to which they do not consent. Still, it is worth keeping in mind that when people consent to be manipulated, they consent to have their behaviour changed in a way that sidesteps their capacity to reflect. They could choose to change their behaviour in a way that makes use of their capacity to reflect.

For further discussion of these issues see Gerald Dworkin, 'Autonomy and Behavior Control', *Hastings Center Report* 6 (February 1976): 23-8.

[15]Feinberg, p. 97.

[16]Nancy K. Janz and Marshall H. Becker, 'The Health Belief Model: A Decade Later', *Health Education Quarterly* 11 (1984): 2-3.

[17]A 'cue to action' is also thought to be important for behaviour change. For instance, personal contact with a person dying from AIDS has been shown to be especially effective in motivating people to adopt low-risk practices (ibid., p. 2).

[18]R.F. Soames Job, 'Effective and Ineffective Use of Fear in Health Promotion Campaigns', *American Journal of Public Health* 78, 2 (1988).

[19]Canadian AIDS Society, *Safer Sex Guidelines* (Ottawa: Canadian AIDS Society, 1989), p. 22.

[20]Canadian Public Health Association, 'The New Facts of Life' (Ottawa: Health and Welfare Canada, February 1988).

[21]Ibid., p. 1 (please note that this brochure is not paginated; the page numbering used here is my own).

[22]Ibid., p. 3.

[23]Ibid., pp. 5-6.

[24]Ibid., p. 5.

[25]Ibid., p. 10.

[26]Ibid., pp. 11-12.

[27]This example is fictitious; it does not reflect the position of the Canadian Philosophical Association.

[28]This was an early campaign of Health and Community Services of the Australian federal government.

[29]Lawrence W. Green, Alisa Wilson, and Chris Lovato, 'What Changes can Health Promotion Achieve and How Long Do These Changes Last? The Trade-offs between Expediency and Durability', *Preventive Medicine* 15 (1986): 516.

[30]Ibid., p. 517.

[31]Ibid.

[32]Ibid., p. 518.

[33]Patricia Illingworth, *AIDS and the Good Society* (London: Routledge, Chapman and Hall, 1990), p. 92; and Ethan Nadelmann, 'The Case for Legalization', *The Public Interest* 92 (1988): 3-31.

[34]Illingworth, pp. 61-102.

[35]Green, Wilson, and Lovato, p. 518.

[36]Ibid., p. 519.

[37]For arguments showing that transmission of HIV is not a harm to others, see Illingworth, pp. 22-60, and Richard D. Mohr, 'AIDS, Gays and State Coercion', *Bioethics* 1, 1 (1987): 35-50 and *Gays/Justice: A Study of Ethics, Society and Law* (New York: Columbia University Press, 1989). Roughly, I argued that with respect to gay men and IV drug users, the transmission of HIV was a self-inflicted harm because it occurred under conditions of consent and in circumstances in which there was not a duty to disclose HIV status.

[38]Robert Allard, 'Beliefs about AIDS as Determinants of Preventive Practices and of Support for Coercive Measures', *American Journal of Public Health* 79, 4 (1989): 448-52.

[39]Richard Titmuss, *The Gift Relationship: From Human Blood to Social Policy* (New York: Vintage Books, 1972).

LIVING WITH AIDS: TOWARDS EFFECTIVE AND COMPASSIONATE HEALTH CARE POLICY

―――――

B. LEE

INTRODUCTION

At the June 1989 Montreal international conference on AIDS, scientists and activists alike presented searing indictments of governmental inaction and incompetence. A visibly nervous Prime Minister Mulroney made his first public speech on AIDS at this conference, eight years into the epidemic.

In contrast to the official record of neglect, there is another side to the politics of AIDS. There is the spectacle of the hundreds of activists who stormed the stage at the Montreal conference to reorder the policy-makers' agenda according to the demands and interests of people living with HIV/AIDS. There is the courage and commitment of PLWAs and the efforts of thousands upon thousands around the world working in the communities most directly affected by the crisis. And there is the amazing history of the transformation of the gay communities of the major cities of North America and Western Europe over the last decade; the rapid restructuring of the sexual and social life of a community under siege.

It is from this side of the AIDS crisis that I will begin. This essay is not so much about why governments have failed so miserably to respond to the

AIDS crisis with compassion and commitment, although this dismal record cannot be avoided. My goal is to sketch out a framework of what social and health policy on AIDS should be; a model of public policy that can both reduce and prevent the spread of infection, and provide the most effective, compassionate, and empowering treatment and care for those living with AIDS.

Most articles on AIDS start with a familiar litany of numbers, with varying degrees of gloom and despair: trends in incidence, epidemiological statistics, projections of cases and costs, etc. I will not repeat the data already presented in the introduction to this book. But some sense of the epidemic's prognosis is a crucial starting point for policy analysis. We do need to know that the incidence of AIDS is bound to increase, depending upon how many uninfected people become infected and how many then become ill; that its impact could be manageable or disastrous, depending upon how rapidly effective treatments are developed and resources committed; and that what does happen in the future will be dramatically influenced by action or inaction now.[1]

I think public policy must be a combination of proactive pessimism (accepting that AIDS may not be eliminated in the immediate future, but striving to reduce the spread of infection and its social and health impact) and dynamic optimism (working for treatment, care, and support that are not just palliative but that enhance the independence and well-being of PLWAs). We cannot simply hope that a cure will one day be found, but must develop treatment and care that see AIDS as a chronic but manageable disease, not as inevitably fatal.[2] We need to redefine AIDS as a crisis that can be prevented and to do so in ways that broaden rather than constrict personal and sexual freedom.

Much of this paper focuses on just what such a policy would look like. The dimensions of the crisis require the mobilization of vast resources, and only the various institutions of the state are in a position to develop and implement the necessary co-ordinated and planned policy. AIDS is the foremost contemporary *challenge* to the resources, commitment, and vision of public policy. How this challenge is met will tell us much about the priorities, values, and assumptions of policy-makers.

The next section looks back on the response to the AIDS crisis to date. Most commentators, from the Royal Society of Canada and leading physicians to AIDS activists and people living with AIDS, argue that the response of governments to the crisis has been ineffective and slow. But at the same time, the energy and imagination shown by the huge numbers of innovative community programs and groups that have emerged in response to the AIDS crisis point the way to policy and programs that could provide the necessary care and support. The third section of this paper will look at how public policy can best meet the challenge of AIDS. If this challenge is met, AIDS could be a *catalyst* for far-reaching changes in the health-care system – reforms that could benefit far more people than those living with AIDS and could enhance the equity and responsiveness of the system as a whole.

LOOKING BACK

Critiques of official policy and programs, not only in Canada but in the United States and Western Europe as well, have come from many quarters.[3] Perhaps most telling of all, activists, advocates, and academics have criticized governments' slowness in responding to AIDS: there was little official attention and even less in the way of resources until the white heterosexual population came to be infected and the 'general population' came to be seen as threatened.[4] This slowness was particularly striking in Western Europe and Canada, where the course of the epidemic was several years behind that in the United States. These governments had the disastrous example of American inaction before their eyes, yet still delayed.

This section cannot be a comprehensive analysis of the nature and basis of state policy and programs on AIDS. Rather, its more modest goals are to set the context for subsequent discussions of policy directions and to identify barriers or obstacles that must be overcome.

State (In-)Action

Official response, when it finally came, was inadequate and inflexible.[5] For example, it was eight years into the epidemic before the Canadian government's regulatory agencies first released desperately needed treatments under the emergency drug-release plan (and then, only under pressure from activist groups and media exposure). Most fundamentally, it was not until June 1990 that the federal government unveiled its long-promised and much-delayed national strategy.[6] This meant, and continues to mean, that the wide range of existing official and community programs, valuable as so many of them are, are not being developed in a planned and integrated fashion.

This lack of coherent strategy has led to a damaging confusion of priorities and directions. One of the most fundamental problems has been a sharp distinction between the traditional public health mandate of preventing the spread of infection, and the treatment and care of the ill and infected.[7] The emphasis in overall health policy has been on the public health part of this dichotomy, protecting the uninfected and combatting the source of infection. By contrast, treatment of the infected and ill has been marginalized as a separate and distinct issue, at best, as lying in the domain of acute or palliative care; at its crudest, the already infected are simply written off.

What has to be seen is the thoroughly political and ideological nature of public health policy.[8] For example, the seemingly laudable concept of protecting the 'general population' screams out that PLWAs, gays, blacks, and other 'high-risk groups' are not part of the rest of society, but a threat that has to be contained or isolated. But public health should not mean solely the protection of the uninfected. The ill and infected are every bit as much part of the 'public' as anyone else, and there has to be a significant increase in the emphasis on treatment and care. What is needed is a reorientation of policy perspectives and assumptions so that the seemingly competing goals of prevention and care can be brought together into a comprehensive and co-ordinated health policy.

Although much expanded in recent years, the scope and content of preventive education and publicity campaigns, and consequently their effectiveness, have been constrained by ideological factors. The initial official campaigns were extremely coy about sexuality, failing to explicitly detail the acts that are dangerous. Current public health campaigns, while perhaps becoming 'sexier', are still framed within messages of abstinence and monogamy.[9] Conservatives continue to attack safer-sex education and condom distribution, believing that this will 'promote' sexual activity, and politicians oppose needle exchanges because they fear being seen as condoning illicit behaviour.[10] These constraints, of course, are hardly surprising. AIDS intersects with contemporary 'moral panics' around sexuality and drugs and the 'New Right' offensive against consensual sexuality.[11]

Significant health-care resources have certainly been devoted to addressing the AIDS crisis, but there are critical institutional barriers to equal access for all PLWAs. Available care remains fragmented between different institutions, disciplines, and settings, confined within a rigid medical division of labour, and provided largely in isolation from community-based services and programs. Medical expertise and resources are also concentrated in relatively few facilities and practices, largely in the major cities. While comprehensive health care is assumed to be available free to all who need it under provincial health plans, many drugs, vitamin supplements, alternative therapies, and other treatments must be paid for individually. Their high cost can be a serious burden for those without drug plans at their workplaces or on low or reduced incomes. As a result of all this, the nature and quality of the care PLWAs receive can vary a great deal.

A further barrier lies in the political economy of biomedical research. While public funds have been available for basic immunological research, the institutional framework of corporate, university, and hospital laboratories 'potentiates competitiveness between clinical investigators, minimizes the sharing of data, and delays the time to the discovery of effective regimens'.[12] In addition, the major pharmaceutical corporations dominate applied research and development, but only drugs that are potentially profitable are of interest to them.

What Needs To Be Done?

The various problems discussed here can have very concrete implications. People can become infected when political opportunism or narrow moralism prevents them from receiving explicit and effective information. People are unable to obtain the comprehensive health care they need because of where they live or how much money they have. People can become ill and die because drugs that may benefit them have not been approved or cost too much. None of this is acceptable in an equitable and compassionate society.

Underlying these obstacles is the failure of federal and provincial govern-ments to take the lead in co-ordinating and funding medical research, devel-oping the full range of necessary treatments, and providing comprehensive and equitable social- and health-support services. That governments have not taken up this leadership role is a clear abdication of their public responsi-bility and a telling indictment of the values and priorities of politicians and policy-makers.

There certainly must be a significant increase in the woefully inadequate public resources devoted to AIDS to date. I will not give a dollar figure for what should be spent on AIDS or a precise outline of necessary programs, for such specifics would quickly become dated. But what is even more impor-tant than a commitment of resources is a transformation of public policy.

Where do we draw this policy from? The most innovative, imaginative, and effective programs have arisen out of the communities most affected by the crisis, especially the gay communities.[13] The guiding principles of a humane and dignified public policy have been forged through the experience of hundreds of community groups and thousands of AIDS activists: respect for individuals' decisions in planning their own health care; equal access to the full spectrum of needed services; a continuum of care that integrates counselling and services and health care and other forms of support; com-munity involvement in the design, operation, and evaluation of all services and programs; and above all else, empowerment of all PLWAs. How to put such principles into practice is the focus of the next section.[14]

LOOKING AHEAD

The magnitude of the crisis and the scale of the resources that will have to be mobilized speak to the need for policy that is sociologically sophisticated and historically informed, flexible and forward-looking, and, most fundamen-tally, whose starting point will be the needs of the ill and infected and of the communities most affected by the AIDS crisis. The following sections flesh out two policy directions: enhanced treatment, care, and support for PLWAs and HIV-positive individuals, and comprehensive and effective preventive programs that can reduce the spread of infection. I will also argue that these two strands must not be arbitrarily separated, but have to be integrated in public policy.

Preventive Programs

The traditional mandate of public-health institutions balances limits on some individuals or groups with the need to protect the overall public from infectious diseases. But the appropriate balance must always be calculated in the context of the specific historical conditions and possibilities of the time and the effect of particular policies on particular communities. For example, contact tracing and the reporting of positive test results to health authorities are assumed to be crucial to preventing the spread of infection. Setting aside the extensive debate about whether such tactics have ever been effective, they can have significant adverse consequences within the particular politics and epidemiology of AIDS. In a context of pervasive heterosexism, considerably heightened by AIDSphobia and the equation of 'AIDS' and 'gay', such policies can increase the vulnerability of PLWAs or the HIV-positive to harassment and discrimination. The fear that their status may be revealed can prevent significant numbers of individuals engaged in high-risk activities from coming forward for the counselling, information, and early treatment that can save their lives, and those of others. The conventional wisdom of public-health policy simply may not work in the specific context of the AIDS epidemic.

Such complexities of the current crisis underscore the importance of learning from earlier public-health campaigns against sexually transmitted diseases. One implication of these earlier efforts is that coercive measures, such as quarantine of infected individuals or perceived 'risk groups', have not been effective in reducing the spread of infection.[15]

Official preventive efforts tend to be directed at the undifferentiated 'general public'. While they may provide basic information about HIV and help to counter prejudice, these campaigns can also result in generalized fear and anxiety rather than behaviour change. They have been criticized for miseducation, for example, in arguing that monogamy is safe, when this depends very much on the past history and current practices of one's partner. Official campaigns are seldom explicit about high-risk activities, and too often simply urge people not to do certain things. For all these reasons, the effectiveness of general educational campaigns in changing individual sexual and needle behaviour would appear to be limited.[16]

By contrast, education and prevention campaigns that arise out of grassroots initiatives aimed at particular groups have far more potential. A recent comprehensive survey found that the effectiveness of preventive programs was not simply a question of clear targeting. More importantly, the needs, preferences, and culture of the particular community must determine the nature of the preventive efforts.[17]

Community programs are also not as limited by moral and political constraints as official programs and institutions are. For example, the efforts that have had a dramatic effect on reducing infection in the gay community have been sexually explicit. As part of a massive mobilization of community support and care, an 'extraordinary effort has been put into public information campaigns in the North American gay communities promoting, not guilt and dread of sex, but individual and collective responsibility for sex and the importance of "safe-sex" practices'.[18] These preventive campaigns arose directly out of a spirited defence of the goals and values of sexual liberation. But if sexual politics have been a factor in the way gay programs have evolved, that is not the only area in which they are important. Broader safer-sex campaigns will not help women if particular sexual cultures and patterns of male domination in heterosexual relations make it difficult for women to negotiate and insist upon the use of condoms, for example.[19] Preventive programs must take account of and, where necessary, directly challenge existing sexual cultures and power relations.

A wide range of preventive campaigns has evolved directly out of specific communities. Prostitutes have organized safer-sex projects in Toronto and other cities, in which sex workers talk with and provide condoms and educational material to other prostitutes. Native, Asian, and black groups have been established in Canadian cities to do educational and support work within their communities. The key point is that programs must be derived from the lived experience of the particular group. So, for example, music and theatre created by and for young people can effectively pass on vital information in understandable ways. Educational efforts also have to go to the places where the risky behaviour actually takes place. This means going to the streets and 'shooting galleries' to reach IV drug users, and employing ex-users in the preventive programs. Preventive efforts can build on existing community resources; for instance, women's clinics or reproductive health centres can be used as places to promote 'safer sex'.

A central goal of public policy must be to encourage and facilitate the often highly imaginative preventive measures that came out of the communities directly affected by the crisis. A pro-active public health policy must build on the strengths of these already established networks and organizations of support and service. This implies significant public funding of and logistical support for community-based programs. This expenditure can be seen as an investment to reduce the far more costly effects, in both human and fiscal terms, of increased infection and illness.

But public investment must not entail centralized control. The potential of community efforts will not be realized if they are stifled by official standards and professionalization.[20] In order to ensure that preventive efforts are relevant to individuals' perceptions and experience and sensitive to community values and needs, the communities themselves must be directly involved in the planning and implementation of all programs and services.

Treatment and Care for PLWAs

PLWAs' most pressing need is for therapies that will control the conditions associated with HIV infection and prevent the onset of full-blown AIDS. In this section I will argue that there is an urgent need for more effective treatments; that care and treatment must be equally accessible to all; that early treatment has great potential; and that the current way in which health care is delivered to PLWAs must be restructured.

Research and Development of More Effective Treatments. The contradictions of the existing system of biomedical research become clear if we consider what the combined resources of the drug companies and government, hospital, and university research facilities would be if they could be co-ordinated to the goal of producing the cheapest and most effective treatment rather than competing for their share of potential markets. In the face of a health emergency like AIDS, this is certainly what must be done. Only the state is in an institutional position to look beyond the immediate interests of profit and markets, and government support for research should be significantly increased. But governments that have seen their role largely in terms of a public health mandate have not taken the lead in co-ordinating corporate and other research or in directly funding applied research.

The problem is not just the level and priorities of funding for applied research, but the framework within which research tends to be organized.[21] Conventional double-blind studies, in which members of the control group receive only placebos, have been criticized as leaving people to die. Existing clinical trials also tend to exclude those who are too ill, or who do not fit the protocols for other reasons, and to under-represent women, minorities, and IV drug users. AIDS advocates have developed the concept of 'catastrophic rights', whereby individuals facing life-threatening situations can choose to take experimental or unproved treatments,[22] and have argued for 'parallel-track' trials. These allow patients access to drugs as soon as safety has been demonstrated (the first and quickest step in the regulatory process) while parallel full clinical trials of effectiveness are still underway.[23]

A vital policy challenge is to combine effective research and development with providing the best treatment, quickly, for PLWAs. A promising direction is offered by Community Research Initiatives (CRIs), which arose in the United States as the gay community and concerned physicians and scientists realized that the major drug companies would never carry out the necessary research. It was CRIs in New York and California that first explored the effectiveness of drugs previously used for other purposes in treating AIDS-related conditions. One of the most significant innovations was the use of aerosolized pentamidine, a preventive treatment that has dramatically reduced mortality from PCP (pneumocystis carinii pneumonia). Initially developed out of the grass-roots CRI movement, this regimen was within a year incorporated into officially approved protocols in the United States.[24] A Community Research Initiative has recently been established in Toronto, with funding from the American Foundation for AIDS Research. Its specific goals are to speed up testing by conducting trials through physicians' offices, expand access to experimental treatments, and enhance community control over research directions and design. It will also co-ordinate its protocols and results with the AmFAR network of forty groups in the United States and Puerto Rico.[25]

Such initiatives seek to investigate all treatments that could benefit PLWAs, not just those that could be profitable to large corporations. They also do not make arbitrary divisions between treatment and research: put most starkly, groups of people are not left to die on placebo treatments as scientific controls. These community initiatives should be funded and encouraged by governments. But such funding should be at arm's-length; public policy must be careful to preserve and facilitate the principles of community control and accountability to PLWAs under which these initiatives have worked.

Equal Access to Effective Treatment. It is not enough to develop better treatments; these treatments must be accessible to all who need them. However, PLWAs face serious institutional barriers within the medical delivery system. Primary-care physicians who care for PLWAs, and hospitals and other facilities that provide treatment, are generally terribly overstretched in the major centres and largely unavailable in other areas. The resources available for primary care must be significantly expanded.

One result of this shortage of resources is that practitioners have great difficulty keeping up with the burgeoning literature on AIDS research and treatment. In response, AIDS activists and service-providers have established treatment registries in a number of Canadian and many American communities to exchange information on the latest protocols, drugs, clinical findings, and trends. The computerization of so many physicians' offices and clinics means that these registries can provide immediate access for any health-care provider to the latest and most comprehensive treatment information. By centralizing research findings and clinical experience they can be a vital means of evaluating which treatments are most promising and which therapies or combinations are best for individuals with particular conditions and symptoms. In April 1990 the federal government agreed to activist demands to establish a national treatment registry.[26]

But such registries are not solely for physicians. They can be resource centres in the broader sense of enabling people to inform themselves of the options available to them and the pros and cons of each. The registries can be one of the means whereby the medicalization of the AIDS crisis is challenged as individuals plan and control their own health care.

It is not enough to facilitate access to the latest information, however; a further crucial barrier is economic. The health-care system is not as universal as commonly assumed, especially for those with chronic illnesses. Most drugs and the wide range of herbal, Chinese, and other alternative therapies actually being used by PLWAs are not covered; and in many cases these costs are incurred at a time when income is already reduced through loss of employment. In addition, a number of drugs have been provided free as part of experimental trials, but their cost will be a huge burden for many if they come onto the market when the trials end (the average dosage of AZT would cost over $400 per month). What may happen is that people will make vital decisions about their health care in terms of cost, contradicting the fundamental principles of equity and universality upon which the health-care system is supposedly based. Governments must not simply add to the drug plans under welfare assistance; this would mean that people have to become impoverished before there is any public responsibility to ensure access to treatment. The better direction is to reform health plans to include the full range of effective therapies, both pharmaceutical and complementary, that PLWAs need free of charge. Only in this way can equal access to health care be ensured.

Early Intervention. As the range and quality of treatments have improved and as more and more clinical experience has been accumulated and assessed, the importance of early intervention has become increasingly clear.[27] Early and aggressive treatment (what is often called accelerated care) can forestall or prevent the development of full-blown AIDS and alleviate the severity of symptoms and conditions. Recognizing this potential, a number of American states have established early-intervention clinics and programs. Initial experience from these clinics would indicate that early intervention can in fact mean lower long-term costs, as well as improved health for the people served.[28] Canadian policy has been notoriously slow to follow these changes.

Continuum of Care

Still, it is not enough to offer earlier, better, and more accessible treatment. An important task is to integrate the services provided by different disciplines, professions, and facilities in a continuum of care covering all the health needs of PLWAs. Such integration makes it possible to avoid duplication and to ensure that nothing is missed in planning an individual's care. For example, networks of primary-care physicians may develop links with other professionals such as neurologists, psychologists, and nutritionists; similarly, special units or committees have been set up within hospitals to co-ordinate related services. But much more is involved than even a thorough reorganization of hospitals and other institutions.

As the various gay community programs expanded early in the epidemic, they began to realize that PLWAs needed many kinds of support beyond the traditional medical sphere. A range of broader programs developed to provide emotional support and help with the day-to-day practicalities of living: social work, financial and legal advice, housing, therapy and counselling, referrals, and overall advocacy with the many agencies and offices with which PLWAs come into contact.[29]

Many kinds of health and other services have been developed or adapted to provide care directly to PLWAs in their own homes and communities. Visiting nurses or other practitioners can change IVs, administer medication, monitor conditions, and provide other care, while cooking, cleaning, and other domestic assistance is provided to people who need it. 'Buddy' systems offer practical assistance and emotional support. Also important to PLWAs wishing to live independently is assisted housing – independent apartments but with different levels of health and domestic support available on-site.

The goal of these programs is to enable people to live as independently as possible in their own homes. This approach responds to people's clear preferences, can give individuals more control over their health care, and is a far more efficient use of resources. Sufficient immediate investment in community programs will mean less demand for far more expensive and inefficient institutional care in the future. If such investment is not made, then more extensive institutional investment will become necessary in years to come. Unfortunately, the record of state policy in taking such a long view has not been good.

To summarize, 'continuum of care' means a comprehensive range of services, both from all the disciplines and professions within medicine and from social, legal, and other support or advocacy services. But this cannot be effective in a piecemeal fashion; the full range of care and support services must be available,[30] and they must be provided in a co-ordinated and integrated manner.[31] This integration must operate not just in terms of good working relationships between the different programs and institutions but, equally importantly, at the level of individual planning – an approach often termed 'case management' – so that all facets of an individual's care and support are planned and co-ordinated. Providing this continuum will require a significant expansion of community-based resources and programs.

The actual mix of programs and services must be based on the precise configuration of needs of particular communities. For example, the changing epidemiology of AIDS means that its impact on specific communities must be carefully considered: gay men (among whom the spread of infection appears to be slowing, but who make up by far the largest number of cases in Canada); IV drug users (among whom incidence appears to be rising and infection could spread rapidly); women (Canada is apparently following the patterns of other countries, with a significant increase in incidence); children infected through perinatal transmission; and women and men infected through heterosexual contact. These patterns all have very different political and public health policy implications. These specific groups and communities will react to infection and illness in very different ways. The provision of vital public services must be adapted to their varying needs and the equally varying resources they have to draw upon. For example, it is crucial to recognize that infection is spreading more quickly in socially disadvantaged groups that do not have the firmly established social and support networks of the gay community and have traditionally not had equal access to the existing health care system.

Community Clinics

A key challenge is to develop policy that can bring together the two themes of a continuum of care and community-based provision of services. One way of doing this is through clinics that both provide a wide range of health and other support services on-site and at the same time are the hub or base from which services to PLWAs in their homes and neighbourhoods are organized and co-ordinated.

Clinics could centralize in one accessible location health and social services that are generally scattered, and provide both clinical treatment and a range of psychological and emotional support services. There could be individual counselling and therapy, support groups, and social and recreational activities, both at the centre and as organized outings. More concrete forms of support could also be available: day care for people who need medical and other assistance throughout the day, respite care for regular caregivers, and meals in a dining area.

The clinics could provide information and referral to other health services and facilities in the area. Clinic staff could be responsible for co-ordinating all of these diverse services provided to an individual and working closely with individuals in planning their care and needs. A further great practical advantage would be that all of an individual's records, both of treatment received at the clinic and elsewhere, and of any follow-up or services provided at home, would be centralized. In these ways the clinics could be the key central locations out of which comprehensive case management is organized.

Community clinics could also play a key role in effective preventive programs. These efforts can be much more than traditional speakers bureaus and condom demonstrations to local schools, clubs, and other groups. For example, projects providing safer-sex education and resources to prostitutes on the streets, or street needle exchanges, could be based at the clinics. Clinics with their roots in local areas and the trust of their communities are far better placed to deliver these types of services than 'official' institutions like hospitals or public health departments.

At best, a network of such clinics should be established, based upon existing resources such as sexually transmitted disease and other clinics, and in turn linked to hospitals, community agencies, hospices, nursing homes, and other relevant programs and facilities.

CONCLUSIONS

To summarize earlier discussions: there must be a significant expansion of health-care resources devoted to HIV; research on the development of effective treatments must be facilitated; PLWAs must have equal access to the full continuum of care and treatment they need; community-based support and preventive efforts must be encouraged and supported; and a vital mechanism to pull all of this together is a network of community clinics.

I have been arguing that we must be concerned not only with what services are available and where they are located and delivered, but also with *how* care is planned, organized, and controlled. This catalogue of vital services means more than a more equitable, effective, and humane delivery of services. The most important impact of these community programs has been to challenge assumptions about *who* should plan and organize health and social support services, and *in whose interests*. The most innovative and responsive programs arose out of the communities most directly affected by the crisis with the explicit goal of empowering PLWAs. How to preserve this community base and extend the goal of empowerment are the key challenges facing public policy.

To meet these challenges will require both increased resources and innovative policy formation. However, the institutional structure of the state itself has been a key barrier to the comprehensive and co-ordinated policy and programs, well integrated into a coherent national strategy, that are required. New policy mechanisms are urgently needed. A number of specific directions, such as a national treatment registry, have been discussed. However, it may be best to centralize responsibility in an independent body, an AIDS council or secretariat not directly located within the administrative structure and corresponding constraints of government departments, but with the mandate, power, and resources to co-ordinate all facets of the public response to the crisis.

A useful model might in fact be to have various levels of AIDS councils – provincial or regional to co-ordinate local efforts and national to enhance overall direction. Whatever national strategy is developed and whatever overall principles come to be shared, they must be adapted to local conditions, interests, and needs so as not to lose the grass-roots character of the most imaginative programs and services that have emerged. This requires a flexible combination of local autonomy and community control with state financial and resource support. It will also necessitate a redefinition of the relation between the state, on the one hand, and the diverse communities affected by AIDS and the networks of support and care they have created, on the other. Public funding of community care, support, and preventive programs must be increased. But this must not serve to increase state regulation of community efforts; rather, it must preserve their independence and responsiveness to PLWAs.

Whatever research, funding, policy, and co-ordinating bodies are developed, a crucial precondition of their effectiveness is that they operate from the standpoint of PLWAs as opposed to corporate profits or state fiscal imperatives. All such bodies must have significant representation from the diverse AIDS community: PLWAs, support and service groups, activists and advocacy groups, health care providers, scientists, other front-line community organizations, and representatives of the social and ethnic groups most affected by the epidemic. The goal would be to have institutions that can mobilize the resources of the state but are still driven by the needs and activism of the communities in the forefront of the crisis.

Even the most effective and compassionate health care policy will still require complementary social, legal, and other policy reforms. For example, the benefits of high-quality neurological care or nutritional counselling are limited if people have just been evicted from their home or have no money to buy proper food. Similarly, people can hardly be expected to come in for antibody testing and counselling if they fear identification and discrimination. Proactive government policy is needed in these cases to improve social assistance and affordable housing and to directly challenge discrimination.[32] Similarly, providing drug users with clean needles and vital preventive and treatment information is extremely difficult in the climate of official surveillance and political timidity that illegality creates. Major obstacles to reaching a group facing a potentially catastrophic rise in infection could be removed by decriminalizing drug use.

We must not be naïve: these policy reforms face powerful obstacles. How can we expect policy-makers and politicians who have failed so miserably in responding to the AIDS crisis so far to make such radical changes? How can we expect an institutional order that plays such a vital role in the maintenance of oppressive relations of power to transform its policies and programs in ways that will empower groups of people who are very much marginal to that power structure? At the risk of being far too simplistic, the answer is that these changes will come about only as a result of significant political pressure. State policy will change only if it is forced to. How to organize the popular support and pressure needed to force these changes is one of the foremost challenges facing the AIDS and other progressive movements today.

If these massive changes in health-care and social policy are brought to pass; if preventive, care, and support programs are established that empower PLWAs, then AIDS could in fact be a *catalyst* for far-reaching changes in health care and social values.

AIDS as Catalyst

It may be difficult, in the midst of such a profound crisis as AIDS, to see the historical significance of how the communities most affected have responded. The way existing services have expanded or adjusted and new services have sprung up to meet the needs of a new health-care crisis has been unparalleled. An even more lasting impact may be the dramatic transformation that has been brought about in the goals and ethos of health care.

First of all, the development of community services, especially in the gay communities, has been based on a far broader concept of health and care. This has meant not just the traditional medical focus on the treatment of symptoms, but the creation of a dense web of social, psychological, housing, financial, legal, and other services that support PLWAs across the entire spectrum of their life circumstances. Second, community-based programs often have explicit goals of providing these services in ways that actually increase individual autonomy and *empower* PLWAs. Rather than services and information flowing one way from the professional provider to the patient, community care is designed to be participatory – to make it possible for PLWAs to play the central role in planning their own health care.

The goal of empowerment has also meant that community programs and groups are concerned with far more than narrowly defined medical issues. For example, as the framing of information and development of programs arose out of the particular culture and demands of specific communities, these services have been offered within a sex-positive and gay-positive context. This is because these programs arose in communities that, having defined themselves through a long struggle for sexual liberation, knew that the AIDS crisis could easily be turned to the advantage of opponents of sexual freedom. The development of safer sex, which must be seen as one of the most dramatic examples of participatory and community health education, recognizes that HIV-positive people and PLWAs continue to be sexual beings. It constitutes a politic and an ethics of sexual behaviour that combines responsibility to protect oneself and others with the eroticization of new practices (or at least, old practices defined in different ways).

On a more prosaic level, the initiatives outlined here that could improve the care and support of PLWAs could also benefit many others. The services and facilities that can support PLWAs, and the lessons to be learned about how to provide them in empowering ways, must also be extended to the elderly, to people with disabilities, and to others with chronic and immune-system illnesses.

Finally, the political struggles that we will need to win to ensure care and support for PLWAs may have a profound social effect. Some ethicists and analysts have stressed the responsibility of all individuals to change their behaviour, not simply to protect themselves, but to protect others. Those individuals who have made significant changes in their needle-sharing and sexual practices certainly have acted for the collective good as well as their own.[33] But there is a further sense of the 'collective' that must be explored. It can also be argued that there is a collective responsibility to provide support and services to the infected and ill. This is pre-eminently a public responsibility of the state, to ensure that comprehensive and compassionate services are equally available to all who need them.

One commentator has argued that the AIDS crisis requires a new social contract: 'It demands that we renegotiate the terms, infusing the contract with an expanded sense of equity – and empathy.'[34] If the struggle for policy and programs that empower PLWAs can be a catalyst facilitating a re-examination and reordering of fundamental societal values, then something significant will have been won from this terrible crisis.

NOTES

I would like to thank Mary Louise Adams, Gary Kinsman, Tim McCaskell, George Smith, Holiday Tyson, Cynthia Wright, and Christine Overall for their criticisms of earlier drafts of this paper.

[1]Richard Goldstein, 'AIDS and the Social Contract', in Erica Carter and Simon Watney, eds, *Taking Liberties: AIDS and Cultural Politics* (London: Serpent's Tail, 1989), pp. 81-94. See also Canada, Parliamentary Ad Hoc Committee on AIDS (Hon. David MacDonald, Chairperson), *Confronting a Crisis* (Ottawa, June 1990), pp. 1-2.

²When we examine the history of medicine and public health policy, especially around STDs and epidemics, we see that the definition of a disease and the discourses that surround it can be as important as its clinical manifestations in shaping policy development. See Elizabeth Fee and Daniel Fox, eds, *AIDS: The Burden of History* (Berkeley: University of California Press, 1988) and Paula Treichler, 'AIDS, Homophobia, and Biomedical Discourse: An Epidemic of Signification', in Douglas Crimp, ed., *AIDS: Cultural Analysis/Cultural Activism* (Cambridge, MA: MIT Press, 1988), pp. 31-70.

³On the United States see Crimp, and Tom Stoddard, 'Paradox and Paralysis: An Overview of the American Response to Aids', in Carter and Watney, pp. 96-106. See other articles in this same collection for the British situation. On Canada see Tim McCaskell, 'AIDS Activism: The Development of a New Social Movement', *Canadian Dimension* 9 (1989): 7-11.

⁴Simon Watney, 'Taking Liberties: an Introduction', in Carter and Watney, p. 28.

⁵See Sandra Panem, *The AIDS Bureaucracy* (Cambridge, MA: Harvard University Press, 1988) on the US. Jeffrey Weeks provides an overview of the changing priorities of state policy on AIDS in 'AIDS: The Intellectual Agenda', in Peter Aggleton *et al.*, eds, *AIDS: Social Representations, Social Practices* (Lewes, East Sussex: Falmer Press, 1989), pp. 1-20.

⁶Canada, Health and Welfare, *HIV and AIDS: Canada's Blueprint*, and the accompanying *Building an Effective Partnership: The Federal Government's Commitment to Fighting AIDS* (Ottawa: Supply and Services, 1990). On the most charitable of interpretations, this was not a national strategy, or even a federal government strategy. It was really only a blueprint for policy development for Health and Welfare, albeit with some hints to other ministries and jurisdictions. It provided no new funding, especially to the community groups that the minister acknowledged have been bearing the brunt of service provision and education; sidestepped crucial issues such as how to ensure that applied research and the development of treatments for people living with AIDS are prioritized; deflected others, such as human rights protection, the availability of condoms, clean needles and adequate treatment facilities in prisons, and immigration discrimination to other ministries; and generally failed to develop concrete and proactive plans for the necessary mobilization of public resources.

⁷George Smith, 'AIDS Treatment Deficits: An Ethnographic Study of the Management of the AIDS Epidemic, the Ontario case', poster presentation at the V International Conference on AIDS, Montreal, June 1989.

⁸For a comprehensive review of the American public health policy response see Ronald Bayer, *Private Acts, Social Consequences; AIDS and the Politics of Public Health* (New York: Free Press, 1989). A key question is how the definitions of 'which public' and 'whose health' are constructed.

⁹Simon Watney, *Policing Desire: Pornography, AIDS and the Media* (Minneapolis: University of Minnesota Press, 1987); Roberta McGrath, 'Dangerous Liaisons: Health, Disease and Representation', in Tessa Boffin and Sunil Gupta, eds, *Ecstatic Antibodies: Resisting the AIDS Mythology* (London: Rivers Oram Press, 1990), pp. 142-55.

[10]Dennis Altman argued that it is a strange morality when it is better to do nothing to prevent the spread of the virus – thus ensuring that more people will become infected and ill – than to explicitly discuss the acts that lead to infection ('The Politics of AIDS', in John Griggs, ed., *AIDS: Public Policy Dimensions* [New York: United Hospital Fund of New York, 1987] pp. 23-33). For a further critique of 'legal moralism' see Dan Beauchamp, 'Morality and the Health of the Body Politic', *Hastings Center Report* (December 1986): 30-6.

[11]A large literature has developed on this intersection: see Jeffrey Weeks, 'Love in a Cold Climate', in Peter Aggleton and Hilary Homans, eds, *Social Aspects of AIDS* (Lewes, England: Falmer Press, 1988), pp. 10-19.

[12]Kenneth Mayer, 'The Natural History of HIV Infection and Current Therapeutic Strategies', in Lawrence Gostin, ed., *AIDS and the Health Care System* (New Haven: Yale University Press, 1990), p. 31.

[13]In his speech releasing *HIV and AIDS: Canada's Blueprint*, Perrin Beatty recognized the tremendous contribution of community activists in the fight against AIDS, and in a very significant departure for the Conservative or any other government, emphasized the leadership of the lesbian and gay community.

[14]I have not addressed a crucial question here. Faced with a health and social crisis of huge proportions, federal and provincial governments have failed on the most charitable of interpretations. Why is beyond the scope of this paper. Key factors to be analysed would be the ways in which AIDS has come to condense a complex of social and sexual anxieties, especially as it was initially seen to be a disease of marginalized or deviant groups; the immediate historical context of the AIDS crisis, especially as it emerged during a period of significant pressure for the retrenchment of welfare state social and health policies and New Right political mobilization; the role of the state in overall 'moral' regulation and the relation of this to pervasive homophobic and conservative sexual ideologies and racism; the historical traditions and mandate of public health policy and the institutional complexity of state policy development; and the political economy of the pharmaceutical industry and the organization of the medical profession. What I do want to emphasize here is that the failures of public policy are not accidental, but reflect quite fundamental facets of the role of the state in contemporary society. This, plus the fact that demands for proactive and empowering policy on AIDS are largely demands on the state for resources or action, means that any analysis of the crisis and of how to respond to it cannot avoid the question of state power. These remain crucial issues for analysts to take up.

[15]Allan Brandt, 'AIDS: From Social History to Social Policy', in Fee and Fox, and *No Magic Bullet: A Social History of Venereal Disease in the United States since 1880* (New York: Oxford, 1987; rev. ed.), especially Chapter 6.

[16]Ronald Valdiserri, *Preventing AIDS: The Design of Effective Programs* (New Brunswick, NJ: Rutgers University Press, 1989), Chapter 5.

[17]Ibid.

[18]Lynne Segal, *Slow Motion: Changing Masculinities, Changing Men* (London: Virago, 1990), p. 162.

[19]Ibid., pp. 164–5; Valdiserri, pp. 162–6.

[20]For an insightful discussion of the potential of community initiatives and the tension with professionalization, see long-time activist Cindy Patton's 'Resistance and the Erotic: Reclaiming History, Setting Strategy as We Face AIDS', *Radical America* 20, 6 (Sept. 1987): 68–78.

[21]See Margaret Hamburg and Anthony Fauci, 'HIV Infection and AIDS: Challenges to Biomedical Research', in Gostin, for an argument that traditional methodology should be more flexible and innovative in response to AIDS-related issues, including 'compassionate' access to experimental drugs.

[22]John Dixon, *Catastrophic Rights: Experimental Drugs and AIDS* (Vancouver: New Star, 1990) and 'Catastrophic Rights: Vital Public Interests and Civil Liberties in Conflict', in this anthology. For an opposing argument supporting established methodology see George Annas, 'Faith (Healing), Hope and Charity at the FDA: The Politics of AIDS Drug Trials', in Gostin.

[23]United States authorities are currently considering approving such trials (*New Scientist* 31 (March 1990) p. 22).

[24]Mayer, pp. 30–1.

[25]*Extra*, 11 May 1990, p. 11.

[26]*AIDS Action News* 10, 24 (June 1990) (Toronto: AIDS Action Now!)

[27]See Mayer, 'Natural History', p. 23. These developments also open the way to seeing AIDS as a chronic manageable disease, as AIDS activists have long been demanding.

[28]Peter S. Arno *et al.*, 'Economic and Policy Implications of Early Intervention in HIV Disease', *Journal of the American Medical Association* 262, 11 (Sept. 1989): 1493–8.

[29]Lewis Katoff and Richard Dunne, 'Supporting People with AIDS: The Gay Men's Health Crisis Model', *Journal of Palliative Care* 4, 4 (Dec. 1988): 88–95.

[30]Carol Levine, 'In and Out of the Hospital', in Gostin, *AIDS and the Health Care System*, pp. 57–60.

[31]The co-ordinated range of programs in San Francisco has been well documented (Mervyn Silverman, 'San Francisco: Coordinated Community Response', in Griggs, *AIDS Public Policy Dimensions*.) Similar developments, although certainly on a smaller scale, have taken place in other cities.

[32]A number of Canadian jurisdictions, including Ontario, have moved to revise human rights codes to specifically address AIDS-related discrimination. American scholars have called for comprehensive national anti-discrimination legislation. Not only could this provide vital concrete legal protection, but it would also have a significant symbolic effect; it would say that PLWAs are a part of the community who must be supported, as opposed to a marginalized danger from whom 'the rest of society' must be protected. See Wendy Parmet, 'An Anti-Discrimination Law:

Necessary, But Not Sufficient,' in Gostin, *AIDS and the Health Care System*, pp. 85–97. For a broader critique of the relation between public health policy and powers and individual rights see her 'Legal Rights and Communicable Disease: AIDS, the Police Power, and Individual Liberty', *Journal of Health Politics, Policy and Law* 14, 4 (Winter 1989): 741–71.

Patricia Illingworth, *AIDS and the Good Society* (London: Routledge, 1990) argues further that not only should discrimination be prohibited, but governments should provide compensation to PLWAs to recognize that the systemic discrimination facing marginalized groups such as gay men and drug users was a factor in their being infected.

[33]Bayer.

[34]Goldstein, p. 93.

SELECTED BIBLIOGRAPHY

Aggleton, Peter, *et al.*, eds. *AIDS: Social Representations, Social Practices*. Lewes, East Sussex: Falmer Press, 1989.

Aggleton, Peter, and Hilary Homans, eds. *Social Aspects of AIDS*. London: Falmer Press, 1988.

'AIDS: The Emerging Ethical Dilemmas'. *Hastings Center Report* 15, 4, Special Supplement (August 1985).

AIDS: A Perspective For Canadians. Summary Report and Recommendations, and Background Papers. Ottawa: Royal Society of Canada, 1988.

Altman, Dennis. *AIDS in the Mind of America: The Social, Political, and Psychological Impact of a New Epidemic*. New York: Doubleday, 1986.

Bateson, Mary Catherine, and Richard Goldsby. *Thinking AIDS*. Reading, MA: Addison-Wesley Publishing Company, 1988.

Bayer, Ronald. *Private Acts, Social Consequences: AIDS and the Politics of Public Health*. New York: The Free Press, 1989.

Boffin, Tessa, and Sunil Gupta, eds. *Ecstatic Antibodies: Resisting the AIDS Mythology*. London: Rivers Oram Press, 1990.

Carter, Erica, and Simon Watney, eds. *Taking Liberties: AIDS and Cultural Politics*. London: Serpent's Tail, 1989.

Corless, Inge B., and Mary Pittman-Lindeman, eds. *AIDS: Principles, Practices, and Politics*. New York: Hemisphere, 1988.

Crimp, Douglas, ed. *AIDS: Cultural Analysis/Cultural Activism*. Cambridge, MA: MIT Press, 1988.

Dixon, John. *Catastrophic Rights: Experimental Drugs and AIDS*. Vancouver: New Star, 1990.

Fee, Elizabeth, and Daniel M. Fox, eds. *AIDS: The Burdens of History*. Berkeley, CA: University of California Press, 1988.

Graubard, Stephen R., ed. *Living With AIDS*. Cambridge, MA: MIT Press, 1990.

Gunderson, Martin, David J. Mayo, and Frank S. Rhame. *AIDS: Testing and Privacy*. Salt Lake City: University of Utah Press, 1989.

Hallman, David G., ed. *AIDS Issues: Confronting the Challenge*. New York: Pilgrim Press, 1989.

Illingworth, Patricia. *AIDS and the Good Society*. London: Routledge, 1990.

King, Alan J.C. *Canada Youth and AIDS*. Kingston, Ont.: Queen's University, 1989.

_____. *Street Youth and AIDS*. Kingston, Ont.: Queen's University, 1990.

Miller, David. *Living with AIDS and HIV*. London: Macmillan, 1987.

Mohr, Richard D. *Gays/Justice: A Study of Ethics, Society, and Law*. New York: Columbia University Press, 1988.

Patton, Cindy. *Sex and Germs*. Toronto: Black Rose, 1985.

Pierce, Christine, and Donald VanDeVeer, eds. *AIDS: Ethics and Public Policy*. Belmont, CA: Wadsworth, 1988.

Price, Monroe E. *Shattered Mirrors: Our Search for Identity and Community in the AIDS Era*. Cambridge, MA: Harvard University Press, 1989.

Richardson, Diane. *Women and the AIDS Crisis*, new ed. London: Pandora Press, 1989.

Rieder, Ines, and Patricia Ruppelt, eds. *AIDS: The Women*. San Francisco: Cleis Press, 1988.

Shilts, Randy. *And the Band Played On: Politics, People, and the AIDS Epidemic*. New York: St Martin's Press, 1987.

Spurgeon, David. *Understanding AIDS: A Canadian Strategy*. Toronto: Key Porter Books, 1988.

Watney, Simon. *Policing Desire: Pornography, AIDS and the Media*. London: Methuen, 1987.

NOTES ON CONTRIBUTORS

H.A. Bassford works in applied ethics, especially professional ethics and health ethics. He is chair of the Department of Philosophy, Atkinson College, York University, and president of the Board of Directors of Casey House Hospice in Toronto, which provides hospice care for people with AIDS.

Jerome E. Bickenbach is an associate professor of philosophy and lecturer in law at Queen's University in Kingston. He currently holds the Bora Laskin National Fellowship in Human Rights Research and is working on philosophical and legal issues relating to physical disablement.

John Dixon teaches philosophy at Capilano College in North Vancouver. He is president of the British Columbia Civil Liberties Association, in which office he has been active in attempting to both formulate and secure the rights of HIV-infected persons. He is the author of *Catastrophic Rights: Experimental Drugs and AIDS* (1990).

Benjamin Freedman is a professor in McGill University's Departments of Medicine, Philosophy, and Humanities and Social Studies in Medicine, and works as clinical ethicist at the Sir Mortimer B. Davis–Jewish General Hospital of Montreal. His areas of research interest include consent, comparative approaches to bioethics, and philosophical and ethical aspects of research with human subjects. His work on the paper in this volume was supported in part by Grant #6605-2897, National Health Research and Development Program of Canada's Ministry of Health.

Patricia Illingworth is an assistant professor in the Department of Philosophy at McGill University. She is also a founding member of the McGill Centre for Medicine, Ethics and Law. Currently on leave from McGill, she is the Senior Ethics Fellow in the Program in Psychiatry and the Law at Harvard Medical School and a Liberal Arts Fellow in Law and Philosophy at Harvard Law School.

B. Lee is a member of AIDS Action Now in Toronto. He also has worked in the Ontario Coalition for Abortion Clinics since 1983 and has written extensively on the politics and practice of the reproductive rights movement.

James Miller, Faculty of Arts professor at the University of Western Ontario in London, teaches an interdisciplinary seminar on AIDS and the arts. He is the curator of 'Visual AIDS', an international exhibition of AIDS posters that has been touring Canada, the United States, and Western Europe since its opening in October 1988.

Christine Overall is an associate professor in the Department of Philosophy at Queen's University in Kingston. She is the co-editor (with Lorraine Code and Sheila Mullett) of *Feminist Perspectives: Philosophical Essays on Method and Morals* (1988), the editor of *The Future of Human Reproduction* (1989), and the author of *Ethics and Human Reproduction: A Feminist Analysis* (1987).

Arthur Schafer is director of the Centre for Professional and Applied Ethics at the University of Manitoba. He is also a professor in the Department of Philosophy and Head of the Section of Bio-Medical Ethics in the Faculty of Medicine.

Michael Yeo is a research associate at the Westminster Institute for Ethics and Human Values in London, Ontario, and teaches ethics at the University of Western Ontario. He has published articles in bioethics and business ethics. His current research interests are in the sociology of applied ethics and in alternative approaches to ethics.

William P. Zion is a professor in the Department of Religious Studies at Queen's University in Kingston. He is the author of *Eros and Transformations: Marriage and Sexuality in Eastern Christian Theology* (1990) and a member of the Board of Directors of the Kingston AIDS Project.

INDEX

WITHDRAWN

No longer the property of the
Boston Public Library.
Sale of this material benefits the Library